BEYOND THE INTERSTATE

DISCOVERING THE HIDDEN AMERICA

Eric Model

WILEY

John Wiley & Sons, Inc.
New York • Chichester • Brisbane • Toronto • Singapore

Publisher: Stephen Kippur
Editor: Katherine Schowalter
Managing Editor: Ruth Greif
Editing, Design, and Production: G&H SOHO
Illustrator: Laura Alexander

This publication is designed to provide accurate and authoritative information in regard to the subject matter covered. It is sold with the understanding that the publisher is not engaged in rendering professional services in the subject matter discussed. Due to the ever changing marketplace, we suggest that you contact the addresses given to verify information.

Library of Congress Cataloging-in-Publication Data

Model, Eric.
  Beyond the interstate.

  Bibliography: p.
  1. United States—Description and travel—
1981- —Guide-books. 2. Festivals—United States—
Guide-books. 3. Holidays—United States—Guide-books.
I. Title.
E158.M83   1989   917.3'04927   88-27862
ISBN 0-471-61389-4 (pbk.)

Printed in the United States of America

89 90 10 9 8 7 6 5 4 3 2 1

ACKNOWLEDGMENTS

With heartfelt thanks to the many event organizers, officials at tourist boards and chambers of commerce, innkeepers, restaurant owners, and others who were so patient when interviewed during the preparation of this book.

Special thanks to Robert Pfeifer, Joseph and Virginia Pfeifer, Robert Sheldon, Laura Alexander and Karen Stark, whose hard work and commitment made a Hidden America database possible.

To Bruce Black, who helped develop the idea of this book, to Katherine Schowalter, my editor, who made the book a reality, and to Lisa Hoving who made it all look and sound so good. Each one's positive disposition made a challenging task more enjoyable.

And finally, to Sylvia and Sidney Model, who have helped in ways too numerous to list. Their lifelong optimism and support, tempered with realism, helped inspire, encourage, and guide this son. I honor them and the values they have maintained.

CONTENTS

Region: South

Spring

Summer

Fall

Winter

Region: Midwest

Spring

Summer

Region: West

Appendix

INTRODUCTION

The title of this book describes it as a guide to "discovering the Hidden America." But one should take a moment to ask just what is meant by the "Hidden America."

It's not likely to be found on a map. Nonetheless, this Hidden America may be found across the land—in Oregon, Vermont, New Mexico, even New York City. It's the individual parts of America that collectively make up the American experience.

It's lobstermen in Maine, loggers at work in the woods of Washington State, a rodeo in Oklahoma, and Blue Ridge Mountain bluegrass. It's the foods, places, peoples, customs, and history that unite Americans, while accounting for the historic diversity that endures to today.

This book and the commitment to help you discover the Hidden America developed from my own personal travels around America. I often searched for, but rarely found, the America that I had read and heard so much about in books and in the media. This quest in search of the Hidden America led me on a journey not only on the road, but in the books, music, foods, and artifacts of America.

In reality, the Hidden America is not much of a secret. It's always been there for the taking. But until recently, many people thought there was little reason to look "beyond the interstate." After all, for many years, travel in America meant heading out to see the U.S.A. in the family car. Especially during the post–World War II and baby-boom years, the car and the superhighway helped thousands of families see America by making previously distant and perhaps mysterious places more accessible. Folks found out that there was more than just the old neighborhood or the "place in the country." A fast drive on a turnpike or thruway to a tourist attraction or national park, with overnight stays at comfortable motels conveniently located on the highway, was the rule (if you were lucky, you might even find a motel room with air conditioning and a television).

1

Today, American travel habits have changed. Relaxation and entertainment are no longer enough. More and more, folks are looking to learn and grow as they travel, not just get away. They are leaving the main roads and exploring the back roads, and visiting inns, quaint hotels, and picturesque towns along the way.

But to find the Hidden America, you must do more than merely follow a back road for a stretch before rejoining the interstate. That is only the starting point. More important than your physical departure from the interstate is your willingness to go "beyond the interstate" in your mind. In fact, this journey of discovery can be taken without ever leaving the comfort of your home. It is an exploration of the literature, the music, the food, the history, and the roots of America, as well as the fruits of "seeing it yourself" through travel.

The focal point for this journey is America's festivals and events. They occur in every corner of the land, throughout the year, and meet all tastes and budgets. They range from the traditional, such as a small-town Fourth of July celebration, to the offbeat, such as the Jumpin' Frog Jubilee.

But America is more than events, and this book is intended to do more than merely provide a list of them. Rather, it is intended to provide insight about the event, about the area, and about the people who make the event significant. Each entry includes a description of the event, a list of local accommodations, recommended places to eat, places of interest in the area, and a bibliography of background readings.

The accommodations included here are those with a "personal touch," in contrast to chain hotels and motels. They range from inns and bed-and-breakfast houses to farms, ranches, and quality hotels. It should be noted, however, that the term "bed and breakfast" means different things to different folks. It is wise to call in advance to be sure that the place described here is the kind of place where you would like to stay.

This book is designed to serve as a sourcebook for discovering the Hidden America. It sets out to assemble and make sense of the scattered information and diverse material dealing with the Hidden America. The result is intended solely as a point of departure and an introduction. My hope is that *Beyond the Interstate* will inform and enlighten its readers—as any good book should—but will also point you in the right direction, armed with enough timely and accurate information so that you can set out on your own personal journey of discovery.

A couple of words of caution are in order.

First, events and accommodations can change without notice. One day's favorite inn may be gone the next. An event traditionally held the third weekend in October may be moved to November or suspended for a year without even a word to the outside world. The information given here was checked before publication, but nonetheless you are strongly advised to call ahead to avoid disappointment.

Because life is not as simple as we would like, noteworthy events do not always occur where inns, bed-and-breakfast places, or quaint hotels may be found. The selection of events for this book has favored those in localities that are well-endowed with accommodations for visitors. In a few cases, however, the nearest accommodations with a "personal touch" are situated an extended drive from the site of the event.

Limitations of space necessitated the exclusion of many worthwhile events and accommodations. In popular areas such as New Orleans, San Francisco, or Cape May, for instance, there are virtually dozens of high-quality places to stay—far too many to list. In addition, there are many festivals and events whose stories still wait to be told. I look forward to the chance to share this additional information at some point in the future.

In the meantime, happy reading and safe, happy journeys.

Eric L. Model
River Edge, N.J.

Key to Accommodation Listings

All information in accommodations listings will appear as follows: Name (type of establishment), address, telephone number; number of rooms, private baths, cost per night; credit cards accepted; children, smoking, disabled, pets, breakfast; host. Description.

Abbreviations

B&B	Bed and Breakfast
I	Inn
H	Hotel
R	Ranch
F	Farm
S	Service
AE	American Express
CB	Carte Blanche
DC	Diners Club
DISC	Discovery
MC	MasterCard
V	Visa
rms	rooms
pb	private baths
ltd	limited
c	children
cc	credit cards
s	smoking
d	disabled
p	pets
h	host
Full Bkfst	full breakfast
Cont Bkfst	continental breakfast
Cont-Plus Bkfst	expanded continental breakfast

EAST

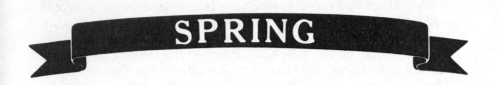

SPRING

Remembering as a Nation

The assembling crowd now stands six deep. The military band that has been playing patriotic march music falls silent. So does the crowd. A military honor guard steps forward and salutes. Taps is sounded. A gun salute is fired.

So starts the annual observance of Memorial Day at Arlington National Cemetery. This gathering and other such gatherings around America maintain a tradition dating back more than a century.

The first Memorial Day was observed in the aftermath of the Civil War. Although the day's exact origins are unknown, Congress credits Waterloo, in upstate New York, as the birthplace of Memorial Day (thought to be in 1866). It was in Waterloo, according to Congress, where a citizen first proposed decorating the graves of fallen heroes. Gradually the practice spread. But other towns—notably Boalsburg, Pennsylvania, which has a tradition dating back to 1864—insist that their memorial observances predate Waterloo's.

Regardless of where the idea first started, the real impetus for an ongoing observance came from veterans of the Union Army. By 1873 their lobbying had succeeded in making Memorial Day a legal holiday in New York, and before long other states followed.

Since the holiday was organized by Union Army soldiers, southern states ignored it. Instead, they observed Confederate Memorial Day. It is still observed in parts of the South. (See "Recalling a Past in Dixie," page 53.)

Memorial Day has become a day of national remembrance for the many thousands of lives lost in all of America's wars. The most recognizable image of Memorial Day is probably the laying of wreaths at Arlington National Cemetery's Tomb of the Unknown

9

Soldier, which contains the remains of people who served in World War I, World War II, the Korean War, and Vietnam. Following the ceremony, there is a memorial service that includes a display of flags, music by the U.S. Navy band, and speeches by leading political and military figures. An audience of some five thousand fills the columned amphitheater; millions more watch the event on television.

While Arlington serves as the traditional focus for Memorial Day observances, some argue that the soul of contemporary observance can be found across the river, at the Vietnam Veterans Memorial.

Designed by Maya Ying Lin and dedicated in 1982, the memorial is a pair of slanting walls of polished black granite, inscribed with the names of the more than fifty thousand Americans killed or missing in Vietnam. Opposite the wall is a more traditional statue of soldiers in combat. Thousands of people visit the site each year. Many leave flowers, letters, medals, pictures, even Army boots, haunting reminders of the pain felt by families and friends.

"It's like a distant bugle that plays silently," explains John Wheeler, chairman of the Vietnam Veterans Memorial Fund. "It pulls people—veterans and nonveterans alike. They come from every part of America."

The memorial presents a striking contrast to the formal white columns at Arlington. "We intentionally sought a spirit of informality and inclusion where people felt comfortable and not in awe," says Wheeler. "To us it's a combination of attitude and setting."

Although the wall initially met with opposition from some veterans' groups, it has become a symbol of healing for the veterans themselves as well as a symbol of their reintegration into the American public, which was for so long unable to come to terms with their suffering. "As the voice starts to become more distant," says Wheeler, "our pain begins to merge. It's less Vietnam War pain, and more a pain common to the tragedy of all war."

The Civil War roots of Memorial Day have long since been merged into a larger observance (the last Grand Army of the Republic parade was held in 1911). But the holiday at the Vietnam Memorial is different.

"It's the voice of the sixties generation being heard," says Wheeler. "It springs from our generation in substance and in style."

Now it's one of the most popular and moving sites in the nation's capital. Wheeler says he knew its success was assured following the first observance at the site in 1980, before construction had begun.

That year, Wheeler invited the public to speak. Each person wishing to participate could say only one thing—the name of a loved one, a friend, or a neighbor who fell in Vietnam.

"The grief that overwhelmed us on the Mall that day somehow was picked up on TV during the news. When we saw the public's response, we knew that the wall had already been built before the workers even showed up to start."

Wheeler continues, "A flame was lit that day. Today it remains an eternal light to the Vietnam vet and the American public."

Event: Memorial Day
When: Last Monday in May
Where: Arlington National Cemetery,
Arlington, Virginia
Vietnam Veterans Memorial, Washington, D.C.

Contact: Military District of Washington
Public Affairs Office
Fort Lesley McNair
Washington, D.C. 20319
(202) 475-0856

Something about the event: America's war dead are honored at the nation's capital. Official ceremonies at the Arlington National Cemetery include a wreath laying at the Tomb of the Unknown Soldier, a memorial service at the amphitheater, and entertainment by the U.S. Navy band. Afternoon ceremonies are held at the Vietnam Veterans Memorial on the mall.

Accommodations with a personal touch:
Kalorama Guest House at Kalorama Park (I), 1854 Mintwood Place NW, Washington, D.C. 20009, (202) 667-6369: 31 rms, 12 pb, $40-80; cc-AE, DC, MC, V; c-over 5, s-yes, d-ltd, p-no, Cont Bksft; h-Tamar Wood. Inn in residential area near Embassy Row and downtown sites. Restaurants and public transportation within easy reach.

Kalorama Guest House at Woodley Park (I), 2700 Cathedral Avenue NW, Washington, D.C. 20008, (202) 328-0860: 19 rms, 12 pb, $40-80; cc-AE, DC, MC, V; c-over 5, s-yes, d-ltd, p-no, Cont Bkfst; h-Barbara Miller. Turn-of-the-century inn features Victorian decor, brass beds, and oriental rugs. Located near Embassy Row, National Zoo, and Metro.

Adams Inn (I), 1744 Lanier Place NW, Washington, D.C. 20009, (202) 745-3600: 17 rms, pb, $35-50; cc-AE, DC, MC, V; c-yes, s-no, d-no, p-no, Cont Bkfst; h-Gene and Nancy Thompson. In Adams Morgan neighborhood, conveniently located but away from the crowds.

Swiss Inn (I), 1204 Massachusetts Avenue NW, Washington, D.C. 20005, (202) 371-1816: 7 rms, pb, $38-48; cc-AE, MC, V; c-no, s-no, d-no, p-no, Bkfst-no; h-Anna Ambuhl. Located two blocks from Convention Center; features convenience and kitchenettes.

Willard Hotel (H), 1401 Pennsylvania Avenue NW, Washington, D.C. 20004, (202) 628-9100: 395 rms, $180-2500; cc-AE, DC, MC, V; c-yes, s-yes, d-yes, p-no, Bkfst-no. Historic hotel (1901) and home to presidents has recently been restored and offers traditional luxury.

The **Jefferson Hotel** (H), 1200 16th Street NW, Washington, D.C. 20036, (202) 347-4707: 100 rms, pb, $75-235; cc-AE, DC, MC, V; c-yes, s-yes, d-ltd, p-ltd, Cont Bkfst. Quality small hotel situated in the middle of town, accessible to everything. Interior features include canopy beds and grandfather clocks.

Roadside food: Washington was once a southern city, and a taste of the South can be experienced at the **Florida Avenue Grill,** 1100 Florida Avenue NW, (202) 265-1586. Included on its menu are buttermilk biscuits, collard greens, chitlins, and ribs. But D.C. is an international city as well. **Old Europe Restaurant and Rathskeller,** 2434 Wisconsin Avenue NW, (202) 333-7600, is an established restaurant that represents the international ambience of the nation's capital. In addition to outstanding dishes such as schnitzel and sauerbraten, it offers a classic European dining atmosphere.

Some readings to enhance travels: Aikman, Lonnelle, *We, The People,* U.S. Capital Historical Society, produced by National Geographic Society, 1978; Lewis, David, *District of Columbia,* Norton, 1976; Federal Writers' Project, American Guide Series, *Washington, D.C.: A Guide to the Nation's Capital,* Hastings, 1968.

Palmer, Laura, *Shrapnel in the Heart, Letters and Remembrances from the Vietnam Veterans Memorial,* Random House, 1987; Bigler, Philip, *In Honored Glory—Arlington National Cemetery: The Final Post,* Vandermere, 1987; Peters, James E., *Arlington National Cemetery: Shrine to America's Heroes,* Woodbine House, 1986.

Turn off here along the way: The **Tomb of the Unknown Soldier** is one of many memorials in the nation's capital. The best known are the **Washington Monument,** on the National Mall at 15th Street NW, (202) 426-6839; the **Vietnam Veterans Memorial,** Constitution

Avenue between Henry Bacon Drive and 21st Street NW, (202) 426-6700; and the **Lincoln Memorial,** West Potomac Park at 23rd Street NW, (202) 426-6841. But there are a number of memorials that are not as well known. They include the **Iwo Jima Statue (Marine Corps Memorial),** Route 50 near Arlington; and the **United States Navy Memorial,** Pennsylvania Avenue between Seventh and Ninth Streets NW, (703) 524-0830. (See also "Independence Day in the Nation's Capital," page 27.)

Event: Town Meeting
When: First Tuesday in March
Where: Waitsfield, Vermont

Contact: Town Clerk
R.F.D. Box 390
Waitsfield, VT 05673
(802) 496-2218

Something about the event: The first Tuesday in March is Town Meeting Day in Vermont. One place where you can see this example of democracy in action is Waitsfield, a quaint town along Route 100 in central Vermont. It is full of inns and near recreation, with a covered bridge just off the center of town.

Accommodations with a personal touch:
   Knoll Country Farm Inn (I), Bragg Hill Road, R.F.D. 179, Waitsfield, VT 05673, (802) 496-3939: 5 rms, pb-no, $30-42; cc-no; c-over 6, s-no, d-ltd, p-no, Full Bkfst; h-Ann Day. Working farm on 150 acres features pond, player piano, and farm breakfast.
   Lareau Farm Country Inn (I), Box 563, Route 100, Waitsfield, VT 05673, (802) 496-4949: 10 rms, 6 pb, $30-45; cc-MC, V; c-yes, s-ltd, d-no, p-no, Full Brkfst; h-Sue and Dan Easley. This 150-year-old farmhouse situated on river provides country accommodations, with pine board floors and country antiques.
   Mountain View Inn (I), Route 17, Waitsfield, VT 05673, (802) 496-2426: 7 rms, pb, $45-65; cc-MC, V; c-yes, s-ltd, d-no, p-no, Full Bkfst; h-Fred and Sue Spencer. This 150-year-old farmhouse became an inn in the 1940s. Old-time ambience includes living room and homemade breakfast.
   Tucker Hill Lodge (I), Route 17, Waitsfield, VT 05673, (802) 496-3983: 21 rms, 15 pb, $58-73; cc-AE, MC, V; c-yes, s-ltd, d-yes, p-no, Full Bkfst; h-Mike Perkins. Fresh flowers and quilts are featured at hillside inn. Also houses four-star restaurant.

Waitsfield Inn (I), Route 100, Waitsfield, VT 05673, (802) 496-3979: 14 rms, pb, $50-70; cc-MC, V; c-over 10, s-ltd, d-no, p-no, Full Bkfst; h-Judy and Bill Knapp. Part of inn dates back to 1825 and features exposed beams, fireplaces, and antique beds. Attached barn was once a parsonage.

Roadside food: The **Common Man**, German Flats Road, Warren, VT 05674, (802) 583-2800. The restaurant occupies an old barn. The menu is Continental and American; specialties are veal and fish. Other restaurants in the nearby Sugarbush ski area include **Sam Rupert's**, Sugarbush Access Road, Warren, (802) 583-2421, which serves pate, veal dishes, fresh fish, and especially good homemade baked breads and desserts; and the **Phoenix Restaurant**, Sugarbush Village, Warren, (802) 583-2777, whose menu is highlighted by sole, lobster, maple pecan chicken, and gourmet desserts that have been described in national culinary magazines.

Some readings to enhance travels: Morrisey, Charles T., *Vermont: A History*, Norton, 1981; Doyle, William T., *Vermont Political Tradition*, Doyle, 1984; Jennison, Keith W., *Vermont Is Where You Find It*, Countryman, 1987; Federal Writers' Project, American Guide Series, *Vermont: A Guide to the Green Mountain State*, rev. ed., Houghton, 1968; Fisher, Dorothy Langfield, *Vermont Tradition: The Biography of an Outlook on Life*, Little, Brown, 1953; Newton, Earl, *The Vermont Story: A History of the People of the Green Mountain State, 1749–1949*, Vermont Historical Society, 1949; Tue, Christine, *How New England Happened*, Little, Brown, 1976; Hill, Ralph N., *Vermont: A Special World*, Houghton, 1969.

Michaels, Greg, ed., *Governments of Vermont*, Municipal Analysis, 1985; Meeks, Harold A., *Time and Change in Vermont: A Human Geography*, Globe Pequot, 1985.

Turn off here along the way: Waitsfield is situated along Route 100, which runs through a valley to the east of the **Green Mountain** range. Once inaccessible, the area has become home to ski resorts, condominiums, and country inns nestled in a traditional New England landscape.

Just to the west of Route 100 is the northern half of the **Green Mountain National Forest**. It provides winter and summer recreation and panoramic views, especially to the west toward **Lake Champlain** and the **Adirondacks**.

March is the tail end of ski season. Area slopes include **Killington, Mad River Glen**, and **Sugarbush**. Cross-country trails include **Mountain Meadows, Mountain Top**, and **Blueberry Hill**.

Event: Patriots Day
When: Third Monday in April
Where: Lexington and Concord, Massachusetts

Contact: Massachusetts Office of Travel and Tourism
100 Cambridge Street, 13th Floor
Boston, MA 02202
(617) 727-3201

Something about the event: The third Monday in April is known today for the annual running of the Boston Marathon. That day was chosen for the race because it is Patriots Day, a legal holiday in the Commonwealth of Massachusetts. Patriots Day commemorates the Battle of Lexington and Concord, which took place on April 19, 1775. It is observed with ceremonies and a reenactment of the battle on Lexington Green. Actors playing Paul Revere and William Dawes redo their famous rides, shouting "The British are coming." They leave the North End of Boston in the morning and arrive in Lexington at 1:30 P.M.

Accommodations with a personal touch:
The **Hawthorne Inn** (I), 462 Lexington Road, Concord, MA 01742, (617) 369-5610: 7 rms, pb, $85-120 dbl; cc-no; c-yes, s-ltd, d-no, p-no, Cont Bkfst; h-Greg Burch. As the name indicates, the site of the inn was once owned by Nathaniel Hawthorne; it was also owned by Ralph Waldo Emerson and Bronson Alcott. Restored home turned inn offers homemade baked goods. It is situated along the historic battle road.
Joan Ashley Bed and Breakfast (B&B), 6 Moon Hill Road, Lexington, MA 02173, (617) 862-6488: 2 rms, pb, $65-75; cc-no; c-no, s-no, d-yes, p-no, Full Bkfst; h-Joan Ashley. In-town bed-and-breakfast near battle site, with gardens and conservatory.
Sterling Inn (I), Route 12, P.O. Box 609, Sterling, MA 01564, (617) 422-6592: 6 rms, pb, $60-75; cc-AE, V; c-no, s-no, d-no, p-no, Cont Bkfst; h-Mark Roy. A turn-of-the-century inn featuring breakfast, lunch, dinner, and sitting area.

Roadside food: Massachusetts is most famous for its New England seafood, but that's over at the ocean, about an hour to the east.
One of the most renowned eateries in New England is the **Wayside Inn** in South Sudbury, Wayside Inn Road, (617) 443-8846. It is known for its colonial-style food.
In Concord, the **Willow Pond** serves up what is described as "down-home" food, including lobster.

Some readings to enhance travels: Murdock, Harold, *The Nine-teenth of April, Seventeen Seventy-Five: Concord and Lexington,* Reprint, 1969 (reprint of 1923 ed.); Tourtellot, Arthur B., *Lexington and Concord,* Norton, 1963; Stein, R. Conrad, *The Story of Lexington and Concord,* Childrens Publishers, 1983; Miller, Penny, *The New England Mind: From Colony to Province,* Harvard University Press, 1953; Mussey, Barrows, *Yankee Life by Those Who Lived It,* Knopf, 1947.

Turn off here along the way: Once you have witnessed the battle reenactment in Lexington, you might stop off at the Visitors Center near the Common, across from the Buckman. There you can obtain a map with directions to the many historic homes and sights around town. They include the Minuteman Statue, the old belfry bell that sounded the alarm to the minutemen, and the burial site of John Hancock.

Over in Concord, the real attraction is the community's famous literary history. Concord was the home of Ralph Waldo Emerson, the inspiring transcendentalist philosopher, and of Henry David Thoreau, whose cabin at Walden Pond is now a major tourist attraction. Louisa May Alcott, Bronson Alcott, and Nathaniel Hawthorne also helped establish the community as a center of progressive thought.

Today this chapter in our history can be experienced at various locations around town. **Emerson House,** on Cambridge Turnpike and Route 2A, (617) 369-2236, served as Emerson's longtime home and now houses his memorabilia, writings, and furnishings. The **Orchard House,** Lexington Road, (617) 369-4118, offers a look at the life of Louisa May Alcott; the **Thoreau Lyceum** at 156 Belknap Street, (617) 369-5912, does the same for the life of Thoreau. A bookstore may be found here too. The three, and Hawthorne, are buried at the **Sleepy Hollow Cemetery** on Bedford Street. Finally, you can try to derive Thoreau-like inspiration at the 500-acre **Walden Pond Reservation,** 1½ miles south of town, where you can visit a replica of Thoreau's cabin.

Event: Maple Sugar Festival
When: Second weekend in April
Where: St. Albans, Vermont

Contact: Chamber of Commerce
P.O. Box 327
St. Albans, VT 05819
(802) 524-2444

Something about the event: This is one of many events that take place in Vermont during the season when the sap runs from the state's maple trees. You can see up close how sap is made into maple syrup by taking one of the sugarhouse tours offered throughout the area, and you can watch competitions for the best flavor, density, and color. In addition to syrup, there is maple fudge, lots of pancakes, music, entertainment, and crafts, including coopering (the making of sap buckets).

Accommodations with a personal touch:
   Berkson Farms (B&B), R.F.D. 1, Enosburg Falls, VT 05450, (802) 933-2522: 5 rms, 1 pb, $25-45; cc-no; c-yes, s-yes, d-no, p-yes, Full Bkfst; h-Richard and Jo Anne Kessler. Mid-19th-century farmhouse situated on a 600-acre working dairy farm. Homegrown and baked foods, antique-filled rooms.
   Johnson House (B&B), 131 Towers Road, Essex Junction, VT 05452, (802) 879-0866: 2 rms, pb-no, $40-45; cc-MC; c-ltd, s-no, d-no, p-no, Cont Bkfst; h-Nancy Johnson. Colonial-style home built on 12 acres with mountain view.

Roadside food: Country-style food is served at the **Lincoln Inn,** 4 Park Street, Essex Junction, VT 05452, (802) 878-3309. Its "country-style" breakfast includes home fries and sausages. The regular menu includes Vermont turkey, baked ham, and baked haddock.

Some readings to enhance travels: Haedrich, Ken, *The Maple Syrup Baking and Dessert Cook Book*, American Impress, 1985; Merriam, Robert L., *Maple Sugar*, Merriam, 1982; Nearing, Helen and Scott, *The Maple Sugar Book: Together with Remarks on Pioneering as a Way of Living in the Twentieth Century*, Schocken, 1971; Perrin, Noel, *Amateur Sugar Maker*, University Press of New England, 1972. (See also "Town Meeting," page 13.)

Turn off here along the way: St. Albans has a colorful history. Located on scenic Lake Champlain, not far from the Canadian border, it has been a stop for smugglers, and even hosted a Confederate invasion during the Civil War (they came through Canada).

Burlington, 25 miles south of St. Albans, is the state's largest city and its capital. Home of the University of Vermont, near the Green Mountains and the Adirondacks and close to Canada, Burlington has become a popular place to relocate—especially for high-tech companies. Highlights in Burlington include the scenic **Battery Park** along the lake and the **Church Street Marketplace.**

Just south of Burlington is the **Shelburne Museum,** Route 7 and Heritage Park, Shelburne, (802) 985-3344. The museum contains one of the nation's largest and most diverse collections of Americana. Items on display range from quilts to a full-sized ship and a reconstructed general store.

Event: U.S. Naval Academy Commissioning Week
When: Third week in May
Where: U.S. Naval Academy, Annapolis, Maryland

Contact: Public Affairs Office
U.S. Naval Academy
Annapolis, MD 21402
(301) 267-3109

Something about the event: Remember the movie *An Officer and A Gentleman?* Well, this is the real thing. The annual rites marking the completion of initial courses at the Naval Academy are highlighted by the traditional Herndon Monument Climb, dress parades, and performances by the Blue Angels.

Accommodations with a personal touch:

Gibson's Lodgings (I), 110 and 114 Prince George Street, Annapolis, MD 21401, (301) 268-5555: 20 rms, 6 pb, $65-120; cc-AE, DC, MC, V; c-yes, s-yes, d-ltd, p-no, Cont Bkfst. Two 18th- and 19th-century buildings furnished in antiques. Situated in historic Annapolis. Limited off-street parking.

Governor Calvert House (I), State Circle, Annapolis, MD 21401, (301) 263-2641: 46 rooms, pb, $120-140; cc-AE, DC, MC, V; c-yes, s-yes, d-yes, p-no, Cont Bkfst. Historic house with restored Victorian rooms.

Maryland Inn (I), 22 Church Circle, Annapolis, MD 21401, (301) 263-2641: 48 rms, pb, $75-105; cc-AE, DC, MC, V; c-yes, s-yes, d-ltd, p-no, Full Bkfst. Historic inn has been operating since the 1700s.

Robert Johnson House (B&B), 23 State Circle, Annapolis, MD 21401, (301) 263-2641; 30 rms, pb, $105-130; cc-AE, DC, MC, V;

c-yes, s-yes, d-yes, p-no, Cont Bkfst. Three historic homes dating back to 1750.

Prince George Bed and Breakfast (B&B), 232 Prince Street, Annapolis, MD 21401, (301) 263-6418: 4 rms, pb-no, $65; cc-MC; c-over 12, s-ltd, d-no, p-no, Cont Bkfst; h-Norma and Bill Grovermann. Antique-filled townhouse in historic Annapolis.

Naomi Reed (B&B), 411 Third Street, Annapolis, MD 21403, (301) 268-4283: 2 rms, pb-no, $32-35; cc-no; c-ltd, s-ltd, d-no, p-no, Cont Bkfst. Old house B&B features period furniture and a porch. Off-street parking. Close to town.

Roadside food: Annapolis is a surprisingly cosmopolitan city that offers a variety of different cuisines. But it remains home to seafood, undoubtedly because of its nautical history and its location along Chesapeake Bay. Soft crabs and crab cakes are two regional specialties. **McGarvy's,** 8 Market Space, (301) 263-5700, and **Rock Restaurant** (formerly Jason's), 400 Sixth Street, (301) 269-0101, are two locations where they may be found. McGarvy's calls its burgers "the best in Maryland." Good food is also served up at **Marmadukes,** Third and Severn, (301) 269-5420, which features crab cakes.

Highly recommended for Sunday morning is a sumptuous brunch at the historic **Maryland Inn** at 16 Church Circle, Annapolis, MD, (301) 263-2641.

Some readings to enhance travels: Bode, Carl, *Maryland,* Norton, 1978; Papenfuse, Edward C., ed., Federal Writers' Project, American Guide Series, *Maryland: A Guide to the Old Line State,* Johns Hopkins University Press, 1976; Miller, Nathan, *The U.S. Navy: An Illustrated History,* American Heritage/Naval Institute Press, 1977; Polmar, Norman, *The Ships and Aircraft of the U.S. Fleet,* 13th ed., Naval Institute Press; Skinner, Michael, *USN: Naval Operations in the Eighties,* Presidio Press, 1986; Smith, Allan E., *Navy Humor and So Forth,* Brunswick, 1985.

Turn off here along the way: Annapolis is the capital of Maryland and possesses quaint streets and renowned colonial architecture. In fact, Annapolis has one of the highest concentrations of 18th-century structures in America. **State Circle,** (301) 268-5576, is the focal point for guided and self-guided tours of the historic neighborhoods, including museums and churches. As you walk through the narrow streets, you feel yourself going back in time, especially down at the foot of the harbor, where slaves brought from Africa were sold to plantation owners.

SUMMER

The Fans They Left Behind

This is a story about baseball, our national pastime. It's also a story about people and neighborhoods, about disappointment, loyalty, and memories of another time. It's about the fans who were abandoned by their hometown clubs . . . fans left behind.

Joe Pfeifer was one such fan. A native of Brooklyn, his team was the Brooklyn Dodgers, affectionately known as "dem Bums." "I grew up listening to Red Barber," he recalls. "It was wonderful. Win or lose, the team brought the whole borough together. The fans, the players, the Dodgers Sym-Phoney [band]—we felt we were all part of a family."

When Joe went to war in the 1940s, the Dodgers were his lifeline to home. "Even when the mails were slow, I always had the Bums through the papers."

"As long as I live I'll never forgive them for what they did to us." The "they" is Walter O'Malley and the Dodgers ownership. In 1956, they transferred the club from Ebbets Field in Brooklyn to Chavez Ravine in Los Angeles. "They broke our hearts," Joe says.

Marty Adler's heart was broken too. Only a kid at the time the team moved west, he began accumulating pictures, autographs, and memorabilia from Ebbets Field. His sidelight soon became a crusade to preserve the legacy and spirit of baseball in Brooklyn. The result was the Brooklyn Dodgers Hall of Fame, now located at the stately Brooklyn Historical Society in fashionable Brooklyn Heights. Here the illustrious past of "the Bums" is recalled, with displays of old uniforms, bats, balls, gloves, street signs, pictures, and newspaper articles. There is also a section devoted to the one-time archrivals of the Dodgers, the New York Giants, who moved from New York in the mid-1950s. In a gesture inconceivable thirty-five years ago, the Dodgers fans now pay tribute to their old rivals.

Baseball fans in other cities have suffered similar fates. In a corner of Boston's New England Sports Museum lies a case of Boston Braves memorabilia. Not many visitors to the museum stop to look. This is only fitting, considering that lack of interest caused the Braves to leave town before the 1953 season.

George Atlison, however, was a loyal Braves fan who grew up two blocks from Braves Field, where he sold hot dogs during the games. "What I most remember is how quiet the crowd was," he recalls. "Braves Field was a large place that looked empty even when fifteen thousand were on hand."

When the Braves moved to Milwaukee, Atlison never lost his affection for the Boston Braves of his youth. For 50 years, he has collected artifacts of the team. "I have a 1914 Braves pennant," he says, "and a Boston Braves schedule for the 1953 season"—a schedule the team never played.

In St. Louis, the old Browns are more popular today than they were back in 1953, when they left town after 51 years. Much of the credit goes to the St. Louis Browns Fan Club, founded and directed by Bill Borst, a university professor of baseball social history. Interestingly enough, Borst grew up in Queens, New York, as a Brooklyn Dodgers fan, and never saw the Brownies play in St. Louis.

The fan club is made up of six hundred members who honor a team that didn't win many ball games (they finished last or next to last 22 times). They were probably best known for fielding a midget (Eddie Gaedel) and a one-armed pitcher (Pete Gray). The fan club holds regular meetings, honors former Browns players, publishes books, sponsors trips to Kansas City to "recapture" the Baltimore Orioles (the former Browns), and runs a Hall of Fame.

Many of the new Browns fans were not yet born in 1953 and never saw them play in their hometown. But old-timers like Chuck Dewitt still remember Sportsman's Park.

"There used to be souvenir stores, hot dog vendors, and saloons in the middle of a residential neighborhood," Dewitt says. "Now the old ball park site is a Boys' Club."

In Philadelphia, there's no official museum or fan club to recall the old Philadelphia Athletics, who moved to Kansas City and then onto Oakland, California. But the Mitchell and Ness Sporting Goods Store at 1129 Walnut Street in Center City is an unofficial A's headquarters.

Mitchell and Ness is one of the few places that still produces authentic old-fashioned baseball uniforms. Old A's players return to the store often to reminisce about the years when Philadelphia was a two-team town.

"Yeah, I remember it," said Bill Eckels. "There used to be bleachers on the roofs of the houses across from the outfield wall. When the A's put up a wall that blocked the view, they just built the rooftop stands higher. Finally, they were disassembled after being declared a fire hazard."

Eckels should know. He used to be fire chief.

Back in the days of the A's, neighborhoods were split between Phillies fans and A's fans. "It wasn't like Chicago where the North Side was for the Cubs, and the South Side for the White Sox," says another longtime fan, Paul Pogharian. "Here every neighborhood had its Phillies fans and its A's fans. On a hot summer's night you would see groups arguing, player against player, which was the better club."

The fans in New York, Boston, St. Louis, and Philadelphia gained new teams to replace the ones they lost. In Washington things were different. Not only did they lose their one team, they lost it twice.

The Washington Senators were most famous for being the hometown favorites in the Broadway show *Damn Yankees*. They were also famous for losing ballgames. The tradition ended in 1959 and again in 1971, when two versions of the Washington Senators moved to Minneapolis–St. Paul and Dallas–Fort Worth, respectively.

Today, after almost two decades of summers without baseball, a Washington Senators Fan Club claims a membership of two hundred. Unlike the fan clubs in New York and St. Louis, the Washington group focuses on the future as much as the past, lobbying to bring baseball back to D.C. In the meantime, there is the annual Old Timer's Game and spring exhibitions played on a football field.

Russ Hodges, the onetime voice of the New York Giants, spoke for many fans after the Giants played their last home game in New York's Polo Grounds. As television cameras scanned the once-proud park, which was soon to be abandoned, Hodges recited the words of Rudyard Kipling's poem "Recessional":

> The tumult and the shouting dies;
>   The Captains and the Kings depart . . .
> Lest we forget—lest we forget!"

Russ Hodges moved with the Giants to San Francisco. But in New York and elsewhere, they never did forget.

Event: Baseball Hall of Fame Induction Ceremonies
When: First weekend in August
Where: National Baseball Hall of Fame, Cooperstown, NY

Contact: National Baseball Hall of Fame
P.O. Box 590
Main Street
Cooperstown, NY 13326
(607) 547-9988

Something about the event: Each year, several former greats of the game are awarded the highest honor in baseball—induction into the Hall of Fame. In recent years, special award categories have been added, including old timers, black players from the old Negro League, and broadcasters and journalists. In addition to the induction ceremonies, two major league clubs square off at Doubleday Field in an exhibition game.

Accommodations with a personal touch:
Hickory Grove Inn (B&B), Route 80, Cooperstown, NY 13326, (607) 547-8100: 4 rms, 1 pb, $55-65; cc-AE, MC, V; c-yes, s-ltd, d-no, p-no, Cont Bkfst; h-Karen and Vince Diorio. A 150-year-old lakeside inn with antique-filled rooms.
Tunnicliff Inn (B&B), 34-36 Pioneer Street, Cooperstown, NY 13326, (607) 547-9611: 17 rms, pb, $60-77; cc-MC, V; c-yes, s-yes, d-no, p-no, Full Bkfst; h-Stewart Cripps. Old inn, which dates back to 1802, was restored in the 1920s and is described as European in flavor. Features are full breakfasts and an old Dutch oven.
Cooper Inn (I), Chestnut Street, Cooperstown, NY 13326, (607) 547-2567: 20 rms, 15 pb, $70-95; cc-AE, MC, V; c-yes, s-yes, d-no, p-no, Cont Bkfst; h-Steve Walker. The inn, like the town, is named after the author, James Fenimore Cooper. The inn is an 1812 structure with antiques, fireplaces, chandeliers, and high windows. Ostaga Resort facilities are available to guests.

Roadside food: The **Crossroads Inn,** Route 28/80, Fly Creek, (607) 547-9804, serves country French cuisine. Specialties include roast duck, rack of lamb, and fresh fish. Cajun is the specialty at the **Dining Room,** 171 Main Street, Cooperstown, (607) 547-2211. Highlights include blackened redfish and crawfish. The **Terrace Cafe,** 10 Hoffman Lane, Cooperstown, (607) 547-8938, serves a Cajun Louisiana Shrimp Diane, Steak Diane in cognac, fresh seafood shipped in daily from Boston, and desserts that include Mississippi mud and grasshopper pie.

Some readings to enhance travels: Bliven, Bruce, *New York,* Norton, 1981; Ellis, David N., *New York: State and City,* Cornell University Press, 1979; Federal Writers' Project, *New York: A Guide to the Empire State,* Oxford University Press, 1940.

Boswell, Thomas, *How Life Imitates the World Series,* Penguin, 1983; Connor, Anthony J., *Baseball for the Love of it: Hall of Famers Tell it Like it Was,* Macmillan, 1984; Barber, Red, *Nineteen-Forty Seven: The Year All Hell Broke Loose in Baseball,* Da Capo, 1984.

Turn off here along the way: In addition to the Baseball Hall of Fame, Cooperstown is the home of the **Farmer's Museum,** S.R. 80, (607) 547-2533, which chronicles the early history of American farming. The museum also features replicas of businesses and offices from America's earlier days, including a general store, doctor's and lawyer's offices, a church, and a print shop.

An outstanding collection of folk art and memorabilia of James Fenimore Cooper may be found at the **Fenimore House,** just east of town on S.R. 80, (607) 547-2533.

Note that a single admission ticket can get you into the Baseball Hall of Fame, the Farmer's Museum, and the Fenimore House.

East of Cooperstown, there is an underground world to be explored at **Secret Cavern** and **Howe Caverns,** (518) 296-8990, where one can find waterfalls and the floor of an ancient ocean 100 to 150 feet below the surface.

To the north lies the **Erie Canal,** built to connect the Great Lakes and the Hudson River, and once one of the wonders of America. Completed in 1825, it still stretches from a point near Albany to western New York State. Although it still navigates vessels through the region, it stands as more of a memorial of another era in American transportation.

Event: Civil War Memorial
When: Last weekend in June
Where: Gettysburg, Pennsylvania

Contact: Gettysburg Travel Commission
35 Carlisle Street
Gettysburg, PA 17325
(717) 334-6274

Something about the event: The Battle of Gettysburg (July 1–3, 1863) was one of the crucial battles of the Civil War and the subject of Lincoln's famous speech. The annual commemoration starts with a parade, followed by a ceremony at the Gettysburg National Cemetery with guest speakers. Flowers are placed on the graves, continuing a tradition started in 1867. Five miles to the south, there is a reenactment of the battle between the Blue and the Gray.

Accommodations with a personal touch:
   Appleford Inn (I), 218 Carlisle, Gettysburg, PA 17325, (717) 337-1711: 10 rms, 2 pb, $75-85; cc-MC, V; c-over 10, s-ltd, d-no, p-no, Full Bkfst; h-Nancy Ordel Gudmenstad. Former mansion turned inn features gourmet breakfasts, antiques in air-conditioned rooms, a sun room, and a parlor with a grand piano.
   Bishop's Rocking Horse Inn (B&B), 40 Hospital Road, Gettysburg, PA 17325, (717) 334-9530: 3 rms, 1 pb, $80; cc-no; c-no, s-ltd, d-no, p-no, Cont Bkfst; h-Karen and Ethan Brown. Inn, a brick and frame house, was a hospital during the Civil War. Situated on a four-acre site, it has a large living room, a brick patio, formal gardens, and a gazebo.
   The Brafferton (I), 44 York Street, Gettysburg, PA 17325, (717) 337-3423: 8 rms, 4 pb, $60-70; cc-MC, V; c-over 7, s-ltd, d-ltd, p-no, Full Bkfst; h-Mimi Agard. Stone structure from 1786 is on the National Register of Historic Places. Street frontage off the Village Green. Behind the doors lie 18th-century vintage antiques, an atrium, a garden, and a mantel that contains a Civil War bullet hole.

Roadside food: Three different periods and cultures converge at Gettysburg. Cuisine based on that of the Civil War era is served up at **Farnsworth House,** 401 Baltimore Street, (717) 334-8838. Game pie is a specialty. For colonial food and ambience, try **Dobbin House,** Steinwehr Avenue, (717) 334-2100. Pennsylvania Dutch food can be found at the **Dutch Cupboard,** 523 Baltimore Street, (717) 334-6227.

Some readings to enhance travels: Davis, William C., *Gettysburg: The Story behind the Scenery,* KC Publications, 1983; Frassanito, William, *Gettysburg: A Journey in Time,* Scribner, 1976; Nitchkey, Charles R., *Gettysburg: Eighteen Sixty-Three and Today,* Exposition Press, 1979.

Turn off here along the way: Gettysburg has historical ties to two presidents.

Abraham Lincoln's famous Gettysburg Address was given at the dedication of the Gettysburg National Cemetery, four months after the battle in which 51,000 lost their lives. Today, the cemetery contains 3,706 graves of soldiers from both the North and the South. The park is marked by more than 1,300 monuments, including one erected by the State of Virginia in memory of Robert E. Lee. Tours are available from the Visitor's Center, S.R. 134, (717) 334-1124.

The other president associated with Gettysburg is Dwight D. Eisenhower. A 230-acre farm in the area was home to the president and his wife, Mamie, and has been preserved. For more information about the **Eisenhower National Historic Site,** S.R. 134, call (717) 334-1124.

In addition to the officially maintained sites in Gettysburg, the town has its share of other tourist attractions, such as a platform overlooking the battlefield.

Event: Independence Day in the Nation's Capital
When: July 4
Where: Washington, D.C.

Contact: Washington, D.C., Convention & Visitors Association
1575 Eye Street NW
Washington, D.C. 20005
(202) 789-7000

Something about the event: The July Fourth celebration in the nation's capital begins with the National Independence Day Parade, which passes many of the monuments on the Mall. In the evening, the National Symphony Orchestra plays a free concert on the steps of the Capitol. The concert is followed by a fireworks show over the Washington Monument.

Throughout the week the Smithsonian Institution holds its annual Festival of American Folklore on the Mall. This unique festival, which showcases the work of artisans, musicians, and crafts workers, honors a different state every year.

Accommodations with a personal touch: See the listings for "Memorial Day," page 11.

Roadside food: See "Memorial Day," page 12.

Some readings to enhance travels: Applewhite, E. J., *Washington Itself: An Informal Guide to the Capital of the United States,* Knopf, 1981; Duffield, Judy, et al., *Washington, D. C.: The Complete Guide,* Random House, 1987; Smith, Jane O., *Washington One-Day Trip Book: One Hundred Offbeat Excursions in and around the Nation's Capital,* EPM Publications, 1984. (See also "Memorial Day," p. 12.)

Turn off here along the way: Any visit to the nation's capital starts with such attractions as the **White House,** the **Washington Monument,** the **Lincoln Memorial,** the **Capitol,** and **Arlington National Cemetery.**

But there's much more than that. For example, the **Corcoran Gallery,** 17th Street and New York Avenue, (202) 638-3211, possesses one of the oldest collections of American art, as well as works by Degas, Rubens, Rembrandt, and Renoir. The **Library of Congress,** First and Capitol Streets, (202) 287-5000, houses some 80 million items in an ornate Italianate Beaux Arts building patterned after the Grand Opera House in Paris. Its copper and marble roof covers a collection that includes three 15th-century Guttenberg Bibles, 3 million pieces of sheet music, 1,500 flutes, and 20 million books. The **National Museum of American History,** part of the **Smithsonian Institution,** Constitution Avenue between 12th and 14th Streets NW, (202) 357-2700, is full of fascinating memorabilia, ranging from the gowns of First Ladies to presidential campaign buttons to locomotives. Highlights include the original star-spangled banner that inspired Francis Scott Key to write the national anthem, sheet music of Irving Berlin's songs, Dorothy's ruby red slippers from *The Wizard of Oz,* Archie Bunker's chair, and, in the lobby, a log-cabin post office, reassembled and still functioning. The museum also features a wonderful gift and bookstore.

Event: Maine Lobster Festival
When: Last weekend in July
Where: Rockland, Maine

Contact: Chamber of Commerce
Box 508
Rockland, ME 04841
(207) 596-0376

Something about the event: Maine's symbol to the world, the lobster, is celebrated at this annual event, which usually takes place the last weekend in July at the Public Landing in Rockland. Calling itself "the Original Lobster Festival," it features crafts, marine exhibits, lobster crate and trap-hauling contests, music, entertainment, and, of course, lobsters and lobster-eating contests.

Accommodations with a personal touch:
   The Belmont (I), 6 Belmont Avenue, Camden, ME 04843, (207) 236-8053: 6 rms, 4 pb, $45-90; cc-AE, MC, V; c-ltd, s-ltd, d-no, p-no, Full Bkfst; h-John Mancarello. Victorian inn is highlighted by quilt-filled rooms and an unusual number of windows (99). It also has a restaurant that serves continental cuisine.
   Goodspeed's Guest House (I), 60 Mountain Street, Camden, ME 04843, (207) 236-8077: 6 rms, pb-no, $35-65 dbl; cc-AE, MC, V; Cont Bkfst; c-over 12, s-no, d-no, p-no. Antique-filled house, 107 years old. Breakfast is served on the outside deck.
   The Swan House (I), 49 Mountain Street, Camden, ME 04843, (207) 236-8275: 5 rms, 1 pb, $55-90; cc-no; c-ltd, s-ltd, d-no, p-no; Full Bkfst; h-Ellen and Herb Jennings. Century-old home, restored as an inn, with panoramic views, situated at foot of state park with hiking paths.
   Whitehall Inn (I), 52 High Street, Camden, ME 04843, (207) 236-3391: 50 rms, 42 pb, $70-130; cc-MC, V; c-yes, s-ltd, d-yes, p-no, Full Bkfst (also dinner); h-Dewing Family. Once the home of a ship captain, the inn overlooks the harbor. The view from the front rocking porch is especially peaceful. Inside, the antique-filled inn features memorabilia of Edna St. Vincent Millay, who once recited her poetry there. New England specialties served from the kitchen.

Roadside food: A Maine institution is the **Lobster Pound,** Route 1, Lincolnville, (207) 789-5550. The seafood is good, but the view and atmosphere are awesome. Another scenic spot is the wharf at Rockport, which is home to the **Sail Loft,** (207) 236-2330.

Some readings to enhance travels: Berner, William, *Maine,* Houghton, 1973; Lee, William S., *Maine: A Literary Chronicle,* Funk and Wagnalls, 1968; Federal Writers' Project, American Guide Series, *Maine: A Guide Down East,* 2d ed., Courier-Gazette, 1970.

Brown, Allen D., *The Great Lobster Chase: The Real Story of Maine Lobsters and the Men Who Catch Them,* International Marine, 1985; Headstrom, Richard, *All About Lobsters, Crabs, Shrimp, and Their Relatives,* Dover, 1985; Pekar, P. M., *How to Build a Lobster Trap,* Rockom, 1986; Taylor, Herb, *The Lobster: Its Life Cycle,* PBL International, 1984.

Turn off here along the way: The Lobster Festival is held in Rockland, but it's really in **Camden,** a few miles to the north, where the true Maine can be experienced. One word of caution, however—this is tourist country, so be prepared. It's very beautiful nonetheless, and well worth the hassles.

Camden is at the western and southern end of the coastal area known as "Down East." The old-time atmosphere can still be felt here. Self-guided walking tours are available. There are not really many "attractions" other than the beautiful scenery and the quaint ambience in town. Boutiques and cafes dot the scene, and a stay down by the dock is always enjoyable.

Lincolnville and the **Camden State Park,** up U.S. 1, offer beautiful views and great seafood.

If you want a quieter scene and have time to spare for a day trip, take the ferry from Rockland out to isolated Vinalhaven Island.

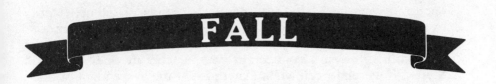

FALL

On Witches, Witchcraft, and Salem

Halloween's always a bit different here. It's a little scarier, a little spookier, the kids a little quieter. But that's to be expected. Wouldn't you feel the same way if you were to spend Halloween in the "home of witches"?

That's how it is in Salem, Massachusetts, site of the infamous witch hunts of the 17th century and the setting for Nathaniel Hawthorne's novel about witch hunting, *The House of the Seven Gables.*

Given its place in American literature and history, it should come as no surprise that officials in Salem treat Halloween as something special. A week's worth of events known as "Haunted Happenings" brings as many as sixteen thousand visitors annually to this city on the north shore of Boston.

One of the oldest cities in New England, Salem was founded in 1626. The witch hunts began in 1692, when a group of teenage girls accused some elderly women of practicing witchcraft. Witchcraft, in the Puritan theocracy, was an offense punishable by death. No defense was possible for the accused. If they insisted that they were innocent, it was taken as proof of their guilt.

Hysteria quickly spread throughout the community. Within a few months, hundreds had been arrested, 19 were hanged, and one man was pressed to death for refusing to enter a plea. Only when accusations were brought against members of prominent families did public opinion turn against the trials. Eventually the girls confessed that they had accused innocent people.

The hysteria over witches that engulfed Salem was not exclusive to that town, says Don Daly of the Essex Institute in town. "It's just that [the Salem witch craze] was the biggest and the last outbreak of witchcraft killings in North America. To a lesser extent it also occurred elsewhere." Indeed, many thousands of women were executed for witchcraft in the British Isles and Europe throughout the premodern era.

Of course, Salem's connection with witchcraft does not end there. It was reinforced when Hawthorne—the descendant of one of the judges at the witch trials—wrote about it in *The House of the Seven Gables*. Today, Salem is the spiritual center of American interest in witchcraft and the occult.

Salem is more than pleased to receive the attention. According to Dan Daly, Salem tried to capitalize on witchcraft as a tourist attraction as far back as the turn of the century. After the loss of its leather industry, Salem used the general fascination with witchcraft to pull itself out of an economic decline. In Salem, they now show off witch images wherever you go—on taxicabs, newspaper titles, road signs, and business signs.

Much of the publicity for Salem has come from transplanted Californian Laura Cabot, who is a self-proclaimed psychic and witch. Cabot claims she knew she was different at three, when she realized she could read others minds. By sixteen, she decided she was a witch and eventually moved to the home of witches, Salem. In the 1970s, she gained noteriety for good-luck incantations for Boston's Red Sox baseball team. Over the vehement objection of the Salem town council, Governor Michael Dukakis designated her as "official witch," and before too long the attractive Cabot could be seen in town attired in black robes.

It soon became known that Laura Cabot was not the only one in town who claimed a religious connection to witchcraft. Today, Salem is said to be home to as many as two thousand witches, in a city of forty thousand people. Cabot is an executive of the Chamber of Commerce. She also acts as a spokeswoman on behalf of witchcraft, appearing in *People Magazine*, and on "The Oprah Winfrey Show," among others. She is out to correct what she believes are misconceptions about witches—especially what she considers "sensational distortions" of witchcraft by the media. "It's going to be a long path and take many years," she says, "but we've been silent too long to the false accusations of those out to do us harm. First we must raise consciousness."

Halloween as it is currently observed in America owes much to the incorporation into Celtic Christianity of pagan practices, including the celebration of a harvest festival on October 31. This festival, called Samhain, is still celebrated by the witches of modern Salem.

Paradoxically, the girls who set in motion the 17th-century witch trials did not live in the city of Salem, but in nearby Old Salem, which shortly afterward changed its name to Danvers. It was not until excavations took place in the mid-1970s that the people of contemporary Danvers found out that their town was the actual site of the accusations (the trials were conducted in Salem).

Even with this revelation, there is little out of the ordinary these days on Halloween for the people of Old Salem (Danvers). They leave all the fuss for Salem and the witches who make their homes there.

Event: Haunted Happenings
When: Last week in October
Where: Salem, Massachusetts

Contact: Salem Chamber of Commerce
32 Derby Square
Salem, MA 01970
(508) 745-1245

Something about the event: Weeklong observance in the city of witches features parades, costume parties, seminars, candlelight tours of a haunted house, and, of course, "real" witches.

Accommodations with a personal touch:
The **Amelia Payson Guest House** (B&B), 16 Winter Street, Salem, MA 01970, (508) 744-8304: 4 rms, 2 pb, $50-75; cc-AE, DISC, MC, V; c-ltd, s-no, d-ltd, p-no, Cont Bkfst; h-Ada Roberts. Greek revival structure from 1845, close to events.

The **Coach House Inn** (I), 284 Lafayette Street (Routes 1A and 114), Salem, MA 01970, (508) 744-4092: 11 rms, 9 pb, $73-80; cc-AE, MC, V; c-yes, s-yes, d-no, p-no, Cont Bkfst; h-Pat Kessler. European-style atmosphere, with Victorian fireplaces and off-street parking.

Salem Inn (I), 7 Summer Street, Salem, MA 01970, (617) 741-0680: 23 rms, pb, $69-90; cc-AE, DC, DISC, MC, V; c-yes, s-yes, d-no, p-no, Cont Bkfst; h-Diane Pabich. Restored Federal mansion in historic district offers antiques, air conditioning, and breakfast in the courtyard garden.

Stephen Daniels House (B&B), 1 Daniels Street, Salem, MA 01970, (617) 744-5709: 5 rms, 2 pb, $85 per day (3-day minimum); cc-AE; c-yes, s-yes, d-no, p-yes, Cont Bkfst; h-Kay Gill. This 300-year-old home turned B&B features antiques, old-fashioned beds, and fireplaces.

Roadside food: Throughout the North Shore region, seafood is the fare. In Salem, it may be had at **Chase House Restaurant**

and Lounge along the Pickering Wharf, (508) 744-0000, where clambakes are arranged. **Finkel's, A Place to Eat,** at 90 Washington Street in Downtown Salem, (508) 745-1630, specializes in seafood and lobsters, as does **Harry's Lobster Shanty** at Salem Market Place, (508) 745-5449, where they serve them up direct from their tanks. The **Lyceum Restaurant** 43 Church Street, Salem, (508) 745-7665, offers history as well. It is where the telephone was first tested. Another seafood hotbed is the **Barnacle Restaurant,** 141 Front Street, Marblehead, (508) 631-4236.

Some readings to enhance travels: Upham, Charles W., *Salem Witchcraft,* 2 vols. Ungar, 1959; Chamberlain, Samuel, *Stroll through Historic Salem,* Hastings, 1969; Boyer, Paul, and Nissenbaum, Stephen, *Salem Possessed: The Social Origins of Witchcraft,* Harvard University Press, 1974; Brown, David C., *A Guide to the Salem Witchcraft Hysteria of 1692,* Brown, 1984; Kent, Zachary, *The Story of the Salem Witch Trials,* Childrens Publishers, 1986; Mappen, Marc, *Witches and Historians,* Kreiger, 1980.

Turn off here along the way: Haunted Happenings features particular events at locations around town. But each of those locations is well worth a visit in its own right. The **Essex Institute,** 132–134 Essex Street, (617) 744-3390, depicts three centuries of history in New England, including textile-making and witch hunts. A ticket to the institute also entitles you to admission to several period homes around town.

The **Peabody Museum of Salem,** at 161 Essex Street on East India Square, (617) 745-9500, houses more than 300,000 objects. They include marine art, ship models, and artifacts from other continents.

Downtown Salem is now a national historic site. Tours of the historic homes and Custom House are available.

Then, of course, there's witchcraft. The **Salem Witch Museum** at 19½ Washington Square, (508) 744-1692, lies opposite Salem Common. The **Witch House** at 310½ Essex Street, (617) 744-0180, was the site of the witchcraft trials. It is open for tours.

Event: Vermont Fall Foliage Festival
When: Late September to early October
Where: Walden, Cabot, Plainfield,
Peacham, Barnet, and Groton, Vermont

Contact: Fall Foliage
Box 38
West Danville, VT 05873
(802) 563-2472

Something about the event: There are quite a few fall foliage festivals around Vermont. But this one is unique. It is a regional festival that moves southward from town to town along with the leaf line. Events include farm tours, band concerts, town dinners, and lumberjack breakfasts.

Accommodations with a personal touch:

Rabbit Hill Inn (I), Lower Wareford, VT 05848, (802) 748-5168: 20 rms, pb, $35-70; cc-MC, V; c-yes, s-yes, d-no, p-yes, Full Bkfst. Country inn in scenic section of Northeast Kingdom. Breakfasts and fireplaces in rooms are highlights.

Nutmaker Inn (B&B), Mountain Road, Box 73, East Burke, VT 05832, (802) 626-5205: 3 rms, pb-no, $30-38; cc-no; c-yes, s-yes, d-no, p-no, Cont Bkfst; h-Lucille Ventres. Cape Cod structure, situated along scenic mountain road.

Highland Lodge (I), Craftsbury Road, Greensboro, VT 05841, (802) 533-2647: 23 rms (11 in lodge, all with pb; 12 in cottage), $75-100; cc-MC, V; c-yes, s-ltd, d-no, p-no, Full Bkfst (also dinner). Lakefront inn with full-sized porch, antiques, brass beds, and traditional furniture. Full dinners of local lamb and chicken.

Roadside food: The area's French Canadian influence is evident at the **Buck and Doe,** Main Street, Island Pond, VT, (802) 723-4712, which serves up pea soup and Gaspe salmon similar to what might be found on the Quebec side of the frontier.

Some readings to enhance travels: Lawrence, Gale, *Vermont Life's Guide to Fall Foliage,* Vermont Life Magazine, 1984. (See also "Town Meeting," page 13.)

Turn here along the way: When visitors turn off the road, it is usually to enjoy the beautiful scenery. But there is civilization here as well. **Cabot** is the birthplace of Zerah Colburn, a mathematical genius and child prodigy. These days, its claim to fame is the **Creamery,** Main Street, (802) 563-2231, where you can see cheese, butter, and cottage cheese being made.

Event: World Pumpkin Federation Weigh-In
When: Second week of October
Where: Collins, New York

Contact: World Pumpkin Federation
14050 Gowanda State Road
Collins, NY 14034
(716) 532-5995

Something about the event: Away for a year in Buffalo, the event has returned to its regular home in Collins. Pumpkin growers from throughout North America, and with an expanded telephone hookup, some international growers—compete. (See "Circleville Pumpkin Show," page 123.)

Accommodations with a personal touch:
   Grape Country Manor (B&B), Old Main Road, Silver Creek, NY 14136, (716) 934-3532: 3 rms, pb-no, $35-45; cc-no; c-yes, s-yes, d-no, p-no, Cont Bkfst; h-Jean Valvo. Sixty-year-old restored colonial home in wooded area. Highlights are antiques and art collection, indoor pool, and sauna. Close to wineries; complimentary bottle of wine served.
   The Teepee (B&B), R.D. 1, Box 543, Gowanda, NY 14070, (716) 532-2168: 3 rms, pb-no, $30-35; cc-no; c-yes, s-yes, d-no, p-no, Full Bkfst; h-Phyllis Lay. Unique experience—B&B located on Indian reservation.

Roadside food: One of the area's favorite eateries is **Waterman's,** 14050 Gowanda State Road, Collins, (716) 532-5995, where the Weigh-in is held. It is a family restaurant featuring chicken and biscuits. Pumpkin pie is served year-round.
   Other area favorites are **Haus Talbick,** on Route 39, in Gowanda, (716) 532-2628, which serves German food, and the **White Inn,** 52 East Main Street, Fredonia, (716) 672-2103, where the highlight entree is called Lamb Wyoming.

Some readings to enhance travels: Gilberg, Richard L., *Pumpkin Cookbook,* Gilmar Press, 1983; Upson, Norma, *The Great Pump-*

kin Cookbook, Maverick, 1984. (See also "Baseball Hall of Fame Induction Ceremonies," page 24.)

Turn off here along the way: Collins is situated in western New York State, just east of the **Cattaraugus Indian Reservation** and in the midst of agricultural and wine country (**Concord Trail**).

The first Farm Grange was founded at **Fredonia** in 1821. Farther to the south lie the Victorian communities of **Westfield** and **Chautauqua,** the world-famous educational and musical enclave.

To the north is New York State's second largest city, **Buffalo.** Once predominantly an industrial city, it is now a financial and cultural hub of the Niagara Frontier. A bit further to the north is **Niagara Falls,** one of the wonders of the world. Though the cities on both the Canadian and the American sides of the falls have become a bit tarnished at the edges since their glory days as a honeymoon destination, Niagara Falls itself is still an awesome sight.

Event: Victorian Week
When: Second week in October
Where: Cape May, New Jersey

Contact: Mid-Atlantic Center for the Arts
P.O. Box 164
Cape May, NJ 08204
(609) 884-5404

Something about the event: Victorian Week celebrates the era when much of Cape May was built. There are tours, period fashion shows, receptions, and a special workshop in restoring old houses.

Accommodations with a personal touch:
The **Chalfonte Hotel** (H), 301 Howard Street, Cape May, NJ 08204, (609) 884-8409: 103 rms, 11 pb, $70–120; cc-V; c-yes, s-ltd, d-ltd, p-no, Full Bkfst (also dinner); h-Ann Leduc. Traditional family hotel dates back to 1876 and features period pieces. (See "Roadside Food.")

The **Queen Victoria** (I), 102 Ocean Street, Cape May, NJ 08204, (609) 884-8702: 11 rms, 7 pb, $59-198; cc-MC, V; c-ltd, s-ltd, d-ltd, p-no, Full Bkfst; h-Joan Wells. Antiques fill this restored 1882 home in the midst of the historic district. There is a Victorian garden.

The **Abbey** (I), Columbia Avenue and Gurney Street, Cape May,

NJ 08204, (609) 884-4506: 7 rms, 4 pb, $58-110; cc-no; c-over 12, s-ltd, d-no, p-no, Cont Bkfst; h-Maryann and Jay Scheffs. Nineteenth-century Victorian one block from beach; afternoon tea is served.

The Main Stay (B&B), 635 Columbia Avenue, Cape May, NJ 08204, (609) 884-8690: 13 rms, 9 pb, $65-110; cc-no; c-over 12, s-no, d-no, p-no, Full Bkfst; h-Sue and Tom Carroll. Built in 1872, inn was once an all-male gambling club. The Italianate villa features Victorian antiques.

Roadside food: The cook of the Chalfonte Hotel has been there for 40 years. The southern-style cooking includes fried chicken, crab cakes, rolls, and biscuits.

Bistros in town include **Louisa's,** 104 Jackson Street, (609) 884-5882, which features seafood and offers a fish pasta dish each night, and **Fresci's,** 412 Bank Street, (609) 884-0366, which also specializes in pasta and seafood. **La Torque,** 210 Ocean Street, (609) 884-1511, offers a varied menu. Highlights are crab soup and roast duck with raspberry sauce.

Some readings to enhance travels: Cunningham, John T., *This Is New Jersey,* Rutgers University Press, 1978; Fleming, Thomas J., *New Jersey,* Norton, 1977; Federal Writers' Project, American Guide Series, *New Jersey: A Guide to Its Present and Past,* rev. ed., Hastings, 1977.

Timmins, Jean Totten, and Parsons, Donald, *This Is Cape May: America's Oldest Seashore Resort,* Timmins Guides, 1985; Gloag, John, *Victorian Taste,* David and Charles, 1980; Dixon, Roger, and Matheius, Stefan, *Victorian Architecture,* Oxford University Press, 1978; Mitchell, Eugene, *American Victorians: Floor Plans and Renderings from the Gilded Age,* Van Nostrand Reinhold, 1983; Landau, Sarah B. and Edward T., and Potter, William A., *American Victorian Architects,* Garland, 1979; Lowndes, Rosemary, and Kailer, Claude, *Make Your Own Victorian House,* Little, Brown, 1981.

Turn off here along the way: Cape May lies at the southern end of New Jersey and is the southernmost resort along the famous Jersey Shore. Beyond the beach, Cape May is distinguished from its neighbors by its late-19th-century Victorian architecture, which is so well preserved that the entire community has been named a National Historic Landmark. To see the quaint town, you can take a guided or self-guided tour. Check the **Information Booth** on Washington Street.

The beach is a favorite spot for making sand castles, fishing, and boating. But of special note are the quartz pebbles, called

Cape May diamonds, that lie on the beach at **Cape May Point.**
The point is also the site of the famous lighthouse that has guided
vessels since 1859. From the lighthouse, you can gaze out toward
Delaware Bay, where you might be able to see the **ferry** that runs
between Cape May and Lewes, Delaware.

Check to see if anything is doing at **Historic Cold Springs Village,**
(609) 884-1810, one-half mile north of the ferry landing. It is a
19th-century farm village that displays crafts and a model South
Jersey farm of the period. Regular and special events are often
scheduled.

Event: Plymouth Thanksgiving
When: Thanksgiving Day
Where: Plymouth, Massachusetts

Contact: Plymouth Area Chamber of Commerce
Memorial Hall
Court Street
Formore, MA 02360
(508) 746-3377

Something about the event: The story of the Pilgrims and their
thanksgiving feast at Plymouth is part of the legend of colonial
America. The annual observance of Thanksgiving at Plymouth
starts with the Pilgrim's Progress, a reenactment of the Pilgrims'
procession to the First Parish Church, where the Thanksgiving
Service is held. A community dinner is served.

Accommodations with a personal touch:
(It is advisable to call in advance because many inns close for
Thanksgiving Day.)
Colonial House Inn (I), 207 Sandwich Street, Plymouth, MA
02360, (508) 746-2087: 7 rms, pb, $60-70; cc-MC, V; c-yes, s-ltd,
d-no, p-no, Bkfst-no. Renovated inn located close to event.
Morton Park Place (B&B), 1 Morton Park Road, Plymouth, MA
02360, (508) 747-2533: 3 rms, 1 pb, $35-65; cc-MC, V; c-ltd, s-ltd,
d-no, p-no, Cont Bkfst; h-Jenine and James Smith. A 130-year-old
New England colonial, situated at park entrance.
Be Our Guest Bed and Breakfast (S), P.O. Box 1337, Plymouth,
MA 02360, (508) 545-6680.

Roadside food: Of course, if you're in Plymouth for Thanksgiving,
the **Town Dinners,** are the place to be for an authentic Plymouth
observance. A community Thanksgiving dinner of turkey and the

trimmings is served at four sittings at Memorial Hall, Court Street. Reservations are required for the dinner (cost is only $16).

A 17th-century Thanksgiving dinner is served at the Plimoth Plantation: S.R. 2A, (508) 746-1622.

Eateries of various types are available. One recommended spot is **Burt's,** 140 Warren Avenue, Plymouth, (508) 746-3422. It features American family-style food and New England lobsters.

McGrath's, Water Street, Plymouth, (508) 746-9751, is a local institution with a colonial ambience.

The **Pilgrim Pantry** on Water Street in Plymouth, (508) 746-4411, still serves up giant clams in traditional style.

Some readings to enhance travels: Applebaum, Diana K., *Thanksgiving: An American Holiday*, Facts on File, 1985; Landis, John T., *Mayflower Descendents and Their Marriages for Two Generations After the Landing*, Genealogical Publishing Company, Inc., 1981; Stratton, Eugene A., *Plymouth Colony: Its History and People, 1620–1691*, Ancestry, 1987; Whitlock, Ralph, *Thanksgiving and Harvest*, Rourke, 1987; Wyndham, Lee, *Thanksgiving*, Garrand, 1963.

Turn off here along the way: Thanksgiving is recalled every day at the historic sites in and around Plymouth. **Plimoth Plantation,** S.R. 2A, (508) 746-1622, is a living museum of 17th-century life where costumed guides practice the gardening, homemaking, and survival skills used by the early Pilgrims. The **Mayflower II**, a full replica of the ship that carried the Pilgrims to America, is moored at the **State Pier,** (508) 746-1622. It is open for touring.

Plymouth contains a number of historic homes, some of which date back to the mid-1600s. They include **Howland House,** 33 Sandwich Street, (508) 749-9590, and **Sparrow House,** 42 Summer Street, (508) 747-1240. Museums that chronicle the story of the Pilgrims and exhibit their artifacts and furnishings include **Pilgrim Hall,** Court and Chilton Streets, (508) 746-1690, and **Harlow Old Fort House,** 119 Sandwich Street, (508) 746-3017, which emphasizes Pilgrim women.

What would Thanksgiving be without turkey and cranberry sauce? You can learn everything you always wanted to know about cranberries at **Cranberry World.** The Visitors Center is on Water Street, Plymouth (508) 747-1000. From there you are taken through working bogs, where you can see harvesting tools and demonstrations.

Thanksgiving comes at the tail end of **whale watch season.** Boat trips leave the Town Wharf, (508) 746-2643.

WINTER

Top Hats and Groundhogs

It all takes place in an instant. We might hear about it on the morning news, then carry on with our business, after being momentarily either encouraged or disheartened by the outcome.

But for the folks of a small Pennsylvania town, this is a most important day, a day that put them on the map.

The town is Punxsutawney, in central Pennsylvania. The event is Groundhog Day. Weather forecasters, townfolk, some tourists, but most of all the news media direct their attention to the reaction of a little furry creature who is bombarded by lights, cameras, and human beings as it leaves its hole. According to legend, if the groundhog sees its shadow on February 2 and hurries back to its underground home in fright, we are in for another six weeks of winter.

How did the legend of the prescient rodent get started? Pennsylvania's earliest settlers were Germans who brought with them an old Scottish couplet that had made its way to Germany from Scotland courtesy of Roman soldiers.

> If Candlemas Day is bright and clear
> There'll be two winters in the year.

When the settlers noticed the profusion of groundhogs in Pennsylvania, they decided that they were most intelligent creatures who should act as the prognosticators of the spring. Accordingly, if on Candlemas Day—February 2—the groundhog saw his shadow and scurried back to his hole, the settlers were willing to take his word for it that there would be a second winter.

According to records maintained in town, it was in the early 1880s that a few citizens of Punxsutawney began to observe the occasion by hying themselves into the woods to honor the groundhog as "the only true weather prognosticator."

41

In 1886, the editor of the Punxsutawney Spirit named this group the Punxsutawney Groundhog Club. It was the nucleus of those who maintain the tradition today. The first official trek to Gobbler's Knob, a hill outside of town and the site of the oracle, was made on February 2, 1887.

For years Gobbler's Knob was closely guarded and closed to the public. Finally, in 1966, the policy was changed. But along with public access came groundhog toys, postcards, golf balls, coffee mugs, license plates, and more. For the centennial celebration in 1987, there was even a special limited edition dinner plate, with groundhog and trim in 24K gold.

Other than the commercial benefits, what does Groundhog Day mean to Punxsutawney?

William Null, director of the Groundhog Day Society, describes an elaborate ritual. According to Mr. Null, the town's groundhog, Punxsutawney Phil, is brought from his heated year-round home at the Civic Center Zoo to a specially heated hole at Gobbler's Knob on the evening of February 1.

On Groundhog Day, the Inner Circle Board of Directors of the Groundhog Club rise no later than 5:30 A.M. to dress in their traditional top hats and tails, as they have for the past 25 years. Then they venture out past town to the Knob.

At 7:30, Jimmy Mears, Phil's handler, will knock on a door to the hole, open it, and ask, "Phil, are you ready?"

Next, according to Mr. Null's account, Phil is "escorted" out. He then starts talking to the club president in Groundhogese, starting with the words "sko sckakapelle," which is alleged to mean "good morning to all." Once the small talk has been concluded, the president becomes aware of Phil's verdict and relays it to the three thousand people present, including those hanging from the trees and the representatives of the news media, who in turn pass it on to the rest of us.

Soon the crowd adjourns to the country club, where a breakfast of eggs, bacon, home fries, coffee, and juice is served. In the evening, they hold the annual banquet. It is unclear whether Phil attends.

Few Americans would dispute Punxsutawney's role as the Groundhog Capital of the World. That is, except for the folks in Sun Prairie, Wisconsin.

There they have come up with their own groundhog, named Jimmy, and made him the archrival of Punxsutawney Phil. They claim that Jimmy is the more reliable rodent—that he's been right something like 23 out of the past 29 years.

The Sun Prairie tradition does not stretch as far back as that in Punxsutawney. The official version has it that in 1948 an artist from nearby Eau Claire suggested that a series of cards be issued through the local post office to commemorate Wisconsin's centennial. One showed a picture of Groundhog Day, and somehow the residents concluded that where better could a groundhog locate its shadow than in a town called Sun Prairie? It was not long before the benefits of this claim were seen by the local Chamber of Commerce. The Chamber designated Sun Prairie the Groundhog Capital of the World, and a legend was born.

A Groundhog Club was started. Anyone born on February 2 was designated a groundhog—everyone else was deemed a woodchuck.

The "tradition" really started to catch on when Sun Prairie decided to take on Punxsutawney as home of the Groundhog. In 1952 the feud was brought to the floor of the United States Congress, when representatives from Wisconsin and Pennsylvania engaged in a heated exchange in defense of their respective groundhog constituents.

Punxsutawney has tried to stay above the fray. It relies upon history and tradition.

Sun Prairie will have no part of it.

They submit that "the shamelessly exaggerated claims of weather forecasting abilities of the Punxsutawney Groundhog have been rightfully exposed." They call Phil a "Jimmy-come-lately" and even have accused Punxsutawney of using a stuffed animal until challenged by Sun Prairie to use the real thing.

Punxsutawney declines to glorify what they consider a frivolous accusation. Instead, they point to the fact that Punxsutawney Phil, not Sun Prairie Jimmy, was invited to the White House by President Reagan a few years back. Mr. Null said the President and the groundhog got along very well.

Event: Groundhog Day
When: February 2
Where: Punxsutawney, Pennsylvania

Contact: Chamber of Commerce
South Gilpin Street
Punxsutawney, PA 15767
(314) 988-7700

Something about the event: Punxsutawney Phil, the clairvoyant groundhog, makes his annual appearance to tell us when spring will arrive. The announcement is made at 7:30 A.M., followed by breakfast. There is a dinner dance later in the day.

Accommodations with a personal touch:
The House of Serian (I), 312 West Mahoning Street, Punxsutawney, PA 15767, (814) 938-3838: 20 rms, 3 pb, $45; cc-no; c-yes, s-yes, d-no, p-ltd, Cont Bkfst; h-Dennis Serian. Historic Victorian mansion with original parquet floors and stairways, and chandeliers in the bathroom.
Gateway Lodge (I), Route 36, Cooksburg, PA 16217, (814) 744-8017; 8 rms, pb-no, $30; cc-no; c-yes, s-yes, d-no, p-no. Log-cabin home in mountains features country breakfast. A drive from the event.
Rest and Repast B&B Service (S), P.O. Box 126, Pine Grove, PA 16868, (814) 238-1484.

Roadside food: There's no groundhog specialty in town. Instead, it's just good food, at spots such as **Ruth and Harry's,** 114 West Mahoning Street, (814) 938-4460, and at the **Panel Hotel,** East Mahoning Street, (814) 938-6600, where one can dine at an enclosed rooftop restaurant.

Some readings to enhance travels: Cochran, Thomas C., *Pennsylvania,* Norton, 1978; Federal Writers' Project, American Guide Series, *Pennsylvania: A Guide to the Keystone State,* Oxford University Press, 1940.
Harris, Mark, *Woodchuck,* University of Georgia Press, 1980; McNulty, Faith, *Woodchuck,* Harper & Row, 1974; Bair, Frank E., and Ruffner, James, eds., *The Weather Almanac,* Avon, 1979; Mitchell-Christie, Frank, *Practical Weather Forecasting,* Barron, 1978; Watts, Alan, *Instant Weatherforecasting,* Dodd, 1968.

Turn off here along the way: One look at the map tells you why they make such a fuss about a groundhog in Punxsutawney. There is not much doing in the area—especially during the winter. Still, there are individual attractions dotting the landscape northeast of Pittsburgh between I-80 and the Pennsylvania Turnpike.
To the southwest is **Worthington's Main Street,** home of the **Old Stone Tavern** at 161 Main Street, (412) 297-3318. It dates back to 1820, when it was a roadside inn. Restored as a museum, it exhibits local crafts.
The railroads have played an important role in the area's history. At **Cresson,** southeast of Punxsutawney on U.S. 22, the **Allegheny Portage Railroad National Historic Site,** (814) 886-8176, recalls the

era when stone was quarried locally for use under railroad ties. The site was also the meeting point of the eastern and western branches of the **Pennsylvania Canal.** A former tavern dating from 1831 hosts a museum that tells the story.

Farther to the east is **Altoona,** founded during the construction of the Pennsylvania Railroad line, a city whose fortunes rose and fell along with the railroad's. The **Railroaders Memorial,** 1300 Ninth Avenue at Station Mall Complex, (814) 946-0835, exhibits trains and memorabilia of railroad history. The **Horseshoe Corner,** a tight bend in the railway line five miles west of town, is an indication of the engineering difficulties that confronted the builders in the mountains.

The line, now operated by Conrail, only hauls freight these days.

Event: First Night
When: December 31
Where: Back Bay and Beacon Hill,
Boston, Massachusetts

Contact: First Night, Inc.
Box 573, Back Bay Annex
Boston, MA 02117
(617) 542-1399

Something about the event: This alternative to traditional, more rowdy, celebrations of New Year's Eve was initiated in Boston in the 1970s. The event centers around cultural events—over 300 of which are available for a single admission price—including ballet, museums, and the symphony.

Accommodations with a personal touch:

Chandler Inn (I), 26 Chandler Street, Boston, MA 02116, (617) 482-3450: 56 rms, pb, $64-74; cc-AE, MC; c-yes, s-yes, d-no, p-no, Cont Bkfst. Inn conveniently located between Park Square and Copley Square.

Copley Plaza (H), 138 St. James Avenue, Boston, MA 02116, (617) 267-5300: 398 rms, pb, $150-210; cc-AE, DC, MC, V; c-yes, s-yes, d-yes, p-ltd, Bkfst-no. Landmark hotel dates back to 1912 and features a four-star restaurant, a wood-paneled bar, and a stately afternoon tea court.

Ritz Carlton (H), 15 Arlington Street, Boston, MA 02117, (617) 536-5300: 279 rms, pb, $175-595; cc-AE, DC, MC, V; c-yes, s-ltd, d-yes, p-yes, Bkfst-no. One of Boston's grand old hotels, with views of Beacon Hill and the Charles River.

Greater Boston Hospitality (S), P.O. Box 1142, Brookline, MA 02146, (617) 277-5430.

Roadside food: Although Boston has traditionally been associated with baked beans, its cuisine is really based on fish. A local institution is **No Name,** 15½ Fish Pier, (617) 423-2705, whose menu includes fresh lobster, scallops, Boston scrod, and their famous chowders. **Anthony's Pier 4,** 1450 Northern Avenue, (617) 423-6363, is another Boston seafood legend. So is **Legal Seafood,** 25 Columbus Avenue, which says it has "the freshest fish served anywhere." Not to be overlooked are the many restaurants in Boston's **North End,** where seafood is given an Italian flavor.

Some readings to enhance travels: Brown, Richard D., *Massachusetts,* Norton, 1978; Chesler, Bernice, *In and Out of Boston With (or Without) Children,* Globe Pequot, 1982; Boston Society of Architects, *Architecture Boston,* Crown, 1976; Howard, Brett, *Boston: A Social History,* Hawthorne, 1976; McIntyre, A. McVoy, *Beacon Hill: A Walking Tour,* Little, Brown, 1975; Blackwood, Alan, *New Years,* Rourke, 1987.

Turn off here along the way: It's unlikely that anyone can come close to seeing all the cultural events that constitute First Night. That leaves much to be seen and done before and after December 31. The best course is to go to the **Greater Boston Convention and Visitors Bureau,** Prudential Plaza, P.O. Box 490, Boston, MA 02199, (617) 536-4100, where you can obtain information about what's doing at these locales (and many others):

For music, try **Symphony Hall,** Huntington and Massachusetts Avenues, (617) 266-1492, home to the **Boston Symphony Orchestra** and the **Boston Pops.** You can also check the **Boston Opera,** (617) 426-5300, and the **Boston Ballet,** at the Wang Center for the Performing Arts, (617) 542-3945 as well as the **New England Conservatory of Music** and several of the city's colleges and universities (including Massachusetts Institute of Technology, Harvard University, and Boston University). Free chamber music concerts are given at the **Isabella Stewart Gardner Museum,** (617) 566-1401.

For art, see the **Museum of Fine Arts,** Huntington Avenue and The Fenway, (617) 267-9377, which contains European, American, Asiatic, and Egyptian works in its permanent exhibits, housed in a structure built in 1909. Its West Wing, opened in 1981, exhibits major traveling exhibitions. The **Institute of Contemporary Art,** 955 Boylston Street, (617) 266-5151, displays 1980s art in a 19th-century structure.

Event: Mummers Parade
When: January 1
Where: Philadelphia, Pennsylvania

Contact: City Representative's Office
Room 1640
Municipal Services Building
· Philadelphia, PA 19102
(215) 686-2876

Something about the event: In this New Year's Day tradition, colorfully costumed Mummers march up Broad Street to the strains of string band music. The festival is an outgrowth of northern European traditions; a southern black influence is evident in the famous Mummers Strut.

Accommodations with a personal touch:
  Society Hill Hotel (I), 301 Chestnut Street, Philadelphia, PA 19106, (215) 925-1919: 12 rms, pb, $85-120; cc-AE, MC, V; c-yes, s-yes, d-no, p-ltd, Cont Bkfst; h-Arlene Mandt. Philadelphia's first urban inn is situated in an 1832 structure and features a piano bar, a restaurant, and Sunday brunch.
  The **Latham Hotel** (H), 17th and Walnut Streets, Philadelphia, PA 19103, (215) 563-7474: 141 rms, pb, $79-155; cc-AE, MC, V; c-yes, s-yes, d-ltd, p-no, Full Bkfst on weekends.
  Bed and Breakfast of Philadelphia (S), P.O. Box 680, Devon, PA 19333, (215) 688-1633.

Roadside food: Philadelphia is a city of culinary legends. At the top of the list is the venerable **Old Original Bookbinders,** 125 Walnut Street, (215) 925-7027, where lobster and seafood are served. It has no connection with **Bookbinders Seafood House,** 215 South 15th Street, (215) 545-1137, which features lobsters, snapper soup, fried oysters and crabmeat.
  Philadelphia tradition is the soft pretzel, which may be purchased at any tourist location. In a pinch, you can make a meal of two pretzels with mustard and a soda. You can see how they are made at the **Philadelphia Soft Pretzel Bakery,** 4315 North Third

Street, (215) 324-4315. It is a little out of the way, but well worth the visit. Call in advance to make sure they save you some pretzels. They go fast.

Some readings to enhance travels: Federal Writers' Project, *Philadelphia: A Guide to the Nation's Birthplace,* Somerset, 1982 (reprint of 1939 ed.); Mease, James, *Picture of Philadelphia,* Ayer, 1970; Llewllyn, Robert, *Philadelphia,* Yankee Books, 1986; Philadelphia Inquirer and Storm, Jonathan, *We The People: A Family Guide to the Constitution City,* Mid-Atlantic, 1987; Sumberg, Samuel L., *Nuremberg Schembart Carnival,* AMS Press, 1941.

Turn off here along the way: The Mummers first surfaced in the mid-1800s, and the parade was added around the turn of the century. You can learn all about them at the **Mummers' Museum,** Second Street and Washington Avenue, (215) 336-3050.

Event: The Great American Chocolate Festival
When: Second weekend
(President's Day weekend) in February
Where: Hershey, Pennsylvania

Contact: Chocolate Festival
Hotel Hershey
Hershey, PA 17033
(717) 533-2171

Something about the event: Heaven for chocolate lovers is Valentine's Day in Hershey, the chocolate city. Chocolate meals are served at the Hotel Hershey. Other features include chocolate-tasting tour, a cocoa bake-off, and a meeting of the Chocolate Lovers' Club.

Accommodations with a personal touch:
   Watsamatter Farm (F), R.D. 4, Box 160, Halifax, PA 17032, (717) 896-3504: 3 rms, pb, $30; cc-no; c-yes, s-yes, d-no, p-no, Full Bkfst. Farm produces milk for Hershey. Property includes a game farm. A 40-minute drive to Hershey and Pennsylvania Dutch country.
   Hotel Hershey (H), P.O. Box BB, Hershey, PA 17033, (717) 533-2171: 254 rms, pb, $122-143; cc-AE, DC, DISC, MC, V; c-yes, s-ltd, d-ltd, p-no, Cont Bkfst-ltd. Hotel and resort are the headquarters for the festival. Amenities such as a sauna and whirlpool are available.

Bed and Breakfast in the Lancaster, Harrisburg, and Hershey Areas (S), 463 North Market Street, St. Elizabethtown, PA 17022, (717) 367-9408.

Roadside food: The **Golden Corral,** 1221 West Chocolate Avenue, Hershey, (717) 533-3699, is known for its steak and a "super salad bar" that includes 160 items. The **Union Canal House Restaurant,** 107 South Hanover Street, (717) 566-0054, offers steak and seafood in a casual family atmosphere. And, don't forget about the All-Chocolate Meal and other meals that feature chocolate as part of the festival at the Hershey Hotel.

Some readings to enhance travels: Asquith, Pamela, *Truffles and Other Chocolate Confections,* Holt, 1984; Boynton, Sandra, *Chocolate: The Consuming Passion,* Workman Press, 1982; Levy, Faye, *Faye Levy's Chocolate Sensations,* HP Books, 1986; Morton, Frederic, and Morton, Marcia, *Chocolate: An Illustrated History,* Crown, 1986; Olney, Judith, *Joy of Chocolate,* Barron, 1982.

Turn off here along the way: True to its reputation, **Hershey** is chocolate town. The name comes from the company's founder, Milton S. Hershey, whose famous product occupies center stage throughout town.

The production of chocolate is the theme of **Hershey's Chocolate World,** Park Boulevard, (717) 534-4900, which demonstrates the entire process, from harvesting cocoa beans in the tropics to packaging the finished chocolate bar in Hershey. Tours are given.

Milton Hershey is honored at **Founders Hall,** S.R. 134 and U.S. 322, (717) 534-3557. His personal memorabilia, as well as displays of Pennsylvania antiques, are highlighted at the **Hershey Museum of American Life,** S.R. 743 and U.S. 422 next to Hershey Park, (717) 534-3439.

If you've had enough of chocolate but are still hungry, you might consider a visit to one of the area's bologna factories. Among them are the **Palmyra Bologna Company,** U.S. 422, Palmyra, PA, (717) 838-6336, and **Bomberger's Bologna,** Fox Road, Lebanon, PA, (717) 273-6794. You learn how the meat is ground, smoked, and packaged. You can continue your culinary tour at the **Sturgis Pretzel Company,** 219 East Main Street, Lititz, PA, (717) 626-4354.

One less publicized but still famous site is the **Three Mile Island** nuclear reactor, Route 441, South Middletown, PA, (717) 367-0518, site of an accident in 1979. They now have a visitors' center, equipped with binoculars that allow you to gaze over to the plant.

SOUTH

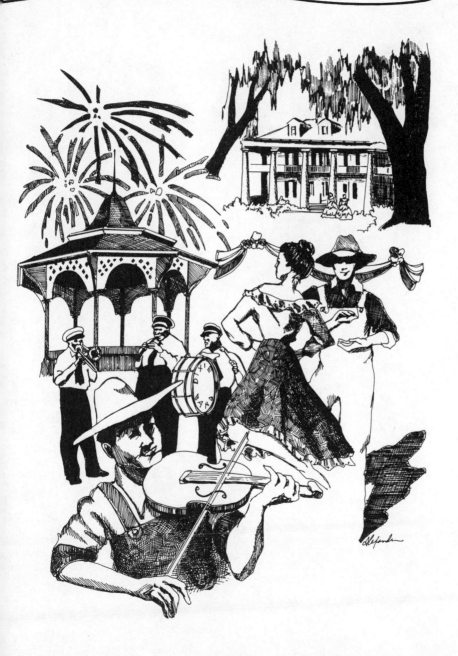

SPRING

Recalling a Past in Dixie

It's a new era in the American South. Covering the land are interstate highways, townhouse developments, shopping centers, corporate parks, and satellite dishes. The trend originated in Atlanta and in the Research Triangle in North Carolina, but it has since spread to Memphis, Louisville, parts of Florida, and a host of other locales as well.

Despite these signs of change, many southerners feel a strong sense of loyalty to the past, and especially to the time when patriotism meant different things in the North and the South.

Nine states of the former confederacy observe Confederate Memorial Day. It's a special time set aside to remember the Confederate Army soldiers who fell in the War Between the States, as southerners call the Civil War.

In Alabama, Georgia, Mississippi, and Florida it is observed on April 26. Other dates are observed in other states: May 10 in North Carolina and South Carolina; May 30 in Virginia; June 3, the birthday of Jefferson Davis, in Louisiana and Tennessee.

The originator of Confederate Memorial Day is thought to have been Elizabeth Rutherford Ellis of Columbus, Georgia. On April 26, 1866, she and a group of Columbus women decorated the graves of soldiers—both southerners and northerners—who had died in local hospitals. In fact, some believe that the "Yankee" Memorial Day was inspired by this one.

Today, Confederate Memorial Day is a legal holiday in Georgia and other states but not all share the same date. However, not many people observe the occasion other than by taking a day off from the routine.

Calvin Johnson is one who does observe it. He is head of the Sons of the Confederacy in Atlanta. He speaks proudly of the many

Confederate Memorial Day ceremonies that take place in Georgia. "We've got to make sure the public doesn't forget," he says. "These men gave up their lives for us."

While some old-timers still look askance at the national Memorial Day (see "Remembering as a Nation," page 9), Johnson, like most southerners, observes both holidays. "I'm proud to be an American and remember the World Wars, Korea and Vietnam," he says. "But I'm also proud of the Civil War dead. We should honor all our ancestors."

Then why not celebrate Confederate Memorial Day on a day that honors all war dead?

"Because the Civil War was different from all the other wars," replies Johnson. "They don't teach about the War Between the States the right way in the schools any more. This observance helps people remember as it should be remembered."

The leaders of the Confederacy are honored on June 3, the birthday of Jefferson Davis, president of the Confederate States of America, West Point graduate, two-time senator from Mississippi, and secretary of state under Franklin Pierce. His birthday is a holiday in Mississippi and nine other states.

The Old Court House Museum in Vicksburg, Mississippi, observes the day with a reception and a public unveiling of Davis artifacts. One year it was a portrait of Davis, another year it was the Davis family's silver and furniture.

At the Rosemont Plantation in Woodville, Mississippi, Jefferson Davis's childhood home, the Davis family holds their annual reunion. Davises come from all over America—even from such Yankee states as New Jersey and New York.

One of the most popular and enduring ceremonies honoring Davis and the Confederacy can be seen at the Vicksburg Memorial Cemetery, where the Daughters of the Confederacy hold a memorial service complete with orators, flowers, and musical performances. Davis's birthday is also observed at the Museum of the Confederacy in Richmond, Virginia, once the Confederate White House.

In many southern states, January 19 is recognized as a holiday in memory of Robert E. Lee, who commanded the southern forces in the War Between the States. Each year his birthday is observed with a convocation at Washington and Lee University in Lexington, Virginia, where he served as president for five years after the defeat of the Confederacy at Appomattox. (See "Confederate Patriots' Birthdays," page 91.)

January 19 is also the birthday of the great civil rights leader Dr. Martin Luther King who, a century after Lee's death, was still fighting the effects of the social system Lee had done his best to preserve. The third Monday in January has been declared a national holiday in his honor.

As the observance of King's birthday has become more widely accepted, the celebrations have become more elaborate. In Atlanta, the event is now a week-long affair based at the Ebenezer Baptist Church. Activities there include a parade, seminars, an ecumenical service, and a community service and banquet.

In Philadelphia, the holiday is commemorated by the symbolic ringing of the Liberty Bell. Honorary ringers have included Benjamin Hooks, of the National Association for the Advancement of Colored People, and Rosa Parks, the woman whose refusal to sit in the "Negroes Only" section of an Alabama bus in 1955 set off a new and dynamic phase of the civil rights movement.

"The King holiday represents us as a nation," says Lloyd Davis of Atlanta's King Center. "How far we have come but how far we still have to go."

Event: Confederate Memorial Day (Georgia)
When: April 26
Where: Various locations in Georgia

Contact: Confederate Memorial Day
Sons of Confederate Veterans
1064 West Mill Drive
Kennesaw, GA 30144
(404) 428-0978

Something about the event: These annual ceremonies, to remember those who fought and died on behalf of the Confederate cause in the "War Between the States," are marked by speeches, flowers, and patriotic music. They are held at the Marietta National Cemetery, the state capitol in Atlanta, the Oakland Cemetery, and the Decatur Court House, among other locations. (Confederate Memorial Day is observed elsewhere in the South, but the date varies from state to state.)

Accommodations with a personal touch:
The **Culpepper House** (I), Morgan at Broad Street, P.O. Box 462, Senoia, GA 30276, (404) 599-8182: 4 rms, pb, $35-60; cc-no; c-yes, s-ltd, d-no, p-no, Full Bkfst. Queen Victoria house, circa 1870, features stained-glass windows and old-time ambience.

Arden Hall (I), 1052 Arden Drive SW, Marietta, GA 30060, (404) 422-0780: 2 rms, pb, $45-50; cc-no; c-no, s-no, d-no, p-no, Full Bkfst. Home turned inn, built in 1880.

Beverly Hills Inn (I), 65 Sheridan Drive N, Atlanta, GA 30305, (404) 233-8520: 17 rms, pb, $59-90; cc-AE, MC, V; c-yes, s-yes, d-no, p-no, Cont Bkfst; h-Lyle Klein. European-style inn features balconies and an authentic London taxi.

Bed and Breakfast—Atlanta (S), 1221 Fairview Road NE, Atlanta, GA 30306, (404) 378-6026.

Roadside food: Dixie cooking is served at **Marymac's Tea Room,** 228 Ponce de Leon Avenue NE, Atlanta, (404) 875-4337. Highlights on the menu include pot likkor, greens cooked with hambone into soup, corn bread, fried chicken, black-eyed peas, and okra, plus other vegetables that change daily. **Aunt Fanny's Cabin,** 2155 Campbell Road, Smyrna, GA 30080, (404) 436-5218, features fried chicken.

Some readings to enhance travels: Coleman, Kenneth, *A History of Georgia,* University of Georgia Press, 1978; Martin, Arnold H., *Georgia,* Norton, 1977; Federal Writers' Project, American Guide Series, *Georgia: A Guide to its Towns and Countryside,* Tubber and Lobe, 1954; Cush, Wilbart, *The Wind of the South,* Random House, 1960; Thorp, Willard, ed., *A Southern Reader,* Knopf, 1955.

Channing, S., *Confederate Ordeal,* Silver, 1983; Clark, James C., *Last Train South: The Flight of the Confederate Government from Richmond,* McFarland & Co., 1984; Jones, Katherine M., ed., *Heroines of Dixie: Confederate Women Tell Their Story of the War,* Greenwood, 1973 (reprint of 1955 ed.); McCardell, John M., Jr., *The Idea of a Southern Nation: Southern Nationalists and Southern Nationalism, 1830-1860,* Norton, 1979.

Turn off here along the way: Stone Mountain is a large dome of granite that measures five miles in circumference and spreads over 583 acres. But look closer and you'll see three large equestrian images of Confederate President Jefferson Davis, Gen. Stonewall Jackson, and Gen. Robert E. Lee. The work took 57 years to complete.

At Stone Mountain Park is the **Antebellum Plantation,** (404) 498-5600, a collection of early-19th-century structures brought from locations throughout the state. They include an overseer's home and slaves' cabins.

The **State Archives,** (404) 656-2393, just east of the state capitol in Atlanta, house many Civil War records. The **Capitol Building** was modeled after the Capitol in Washington.

History abounds in the area surrounding Atlanta. **Kennesaw** was the site of a major Civil War battle. Earthworks from that time have been preserved at the **Kennesaw National Battlefield Monument** north of Stylesboro Road & Old Route 41 intersection, Marietta, (404) 427-4686.

One of the annual ceremonies for Confederate Memorial Day is held at the **Marietta National Cemetery**, (404) 428-5631. A local businessman donated land so that the dead of North and South could be interred. But bitterness was so pervasive that the burials had to occur in separate locations.

Event: National Whistlers' Convention
When: Last weekend in April
Where: Louisburg, North Carolina

Contact: Franklin County Arts Council
P.O. Box 758
Louisburg, NC 27549
(919) 496-2521, ext. 226

Something about the event: The oldest Whistlers' Convention in the nation brings together professionals and amateurs from throughout the country. There are contests, concerts, and workshops. Prizes are awarded to the loudest, oldest, and youngest whistlers. Categories include classical, contemporary, and novelty music. The country's only Whistlers' Museum also displays articles on, and objects connected with, whistles and whistlers.

Accommodations with a personal touch:
The **Oakwood Inn** (I), 411 North Bloodworth Street, Raleigh, NC 27604, (919) 832-9712: 6 rms, 2 pb, $55-65, cc-MC, V; c-over 12, s-yes, d-no, p-no, Full Bkfst; h-Diana Newton. Period Victorian antiques are just one of the features at this 1871 inn, which is on the National Register of Historic Places.

Kings Arm Inn (I), 212 Pollack Street, P.O. Box 1085, New Bern, NC 28560, (919) 638-4409: 9 rms, pb, $52-58, cc-AE, MC, V; c-yes, s-yes, d-yes, p-no, Full Bkfst; h-Barbara and Jerry Ryan. Restored 1775 colonial home turned B&B on former plantation features needlepoint, piano, and homemade food.

Roadside food: This is indisputably barbecue country, with many barbecue drive-ins and pits. At the top of many lists is **Bullicks BBQ,** 3330 Wortham Street, Durham, (919) 383-3211. In addition to classic southern barbecue, it also serves Brunswick stew.

Some readings to enhance travels: Lefler, Hugh T., *North Carolina: The Story of a Southern State,* University of North Carolina Press, 1973; Powell, William S., *North Carolina,* Norton, 1977; Federal Writers' Project, American Guide Series, *North Carolina: A Guide to the Old North State,* rev. ed., University of North Carolina Press, 1955.

Brandon, Jim, *Weird America,* Dutton, 1978; Davidson, Jim, *An Eccentric Guide to the United States,* Berkley, 1977; Stern, Jane, *Amazing America,* Random House, 1978.

Turn off here along the way: Louisburg is located between Interstates 85 and 95, making it easy for visitors to discover North Carolina's diversity. To the east lies the lowland, near the ocean. To the west are the Blue Ridge and Piedmont mountains. The state's central area has undergone a boom in recent years and has changed from farmland into a megalopolis.

The area's growth was spurred by the development of the **Research Triangle,** highly favored by corporations, which draw on the resources of three local universities—the University of North Carolina, North Carolina State, and Duke. The cities of the central area have their own identities: Greensboro is a corporation city, Winston-Salem and Durham are tobacco towns, and Raleigh is the state capital.

Some attractions of special note include the **North Carolina Museum of History,** 109 East Jones Street, Raleigh, (919) 733-3894, which traces art and culture from the colonies to today; **Discover Place,** 301 North Tryon Street, Charlotte, (704) 372-6761, a contemporary science museum featuring a three-story tropical rain forest and a science circus; the **Duke Gardens,** on the west campus of Duke University, Durham, (919) 684-3698; and **Heritage Village,** Business Highway 21, Fort Hills, SC, (704) 544-8100, a theme park that used to be the showpiece of Jim and Tammy Baker's PTL Movement (take I-77 to exit 74).

Winston-Salem goes back to 1766, when Salem was settled by the Moravians (Winston was settled in 1849). The two cities, both centers of the tobacco industry, merged in 1913. You can visit the restored **Moravian Village,** where tours of nine of the 63 restored buildings are available. For information, contact the Old Salem Visitors Center, Old Salem Road, Winston-Salem, (919) 723-3688.

Event: Catfish Capital of the World Festival
When: First Saturday in April
Where: Belzoni, Mississippi

Contact: Catfish Festival
P.O. Box 268
Belzoni, MS 39038
(601) 247-2616

Something about the event: Catfish is king in the Mississippi Delta. Here it is celebrated with entertainment, a pageant, sports, catfish dinners, and a catfish-eating contest.

Accommodations with a personal touch:
   Anchua (I), 1010 East First Street, Vicksburg, MS 39180, (601) 636-4931: 9 rms, pb, $75-105; cc-AE, DISC, MC, V; c-yes, s-yes, d-no, p-ltd, Full Bkfst; h-Kathy Tanner. Greek Revival mansion from 1830 still uses gas burning chandeliers. Period antiques.
   Grey Oaks (I), 4141 Rifle Range Road, Vicksburg, MS 39180, (601) 638-3690: 3 rms, 3 pb, $75; cc-MC, V; c-over 12, s-no, d-ltd, p-no, Cont-Plus Bkfst; h-Ann Hall. Mansion is a replica of Tara from *Gone with the Wind.*
   Cedar Grove Mansion (I), 2200 Oak Street, Vicksburg, MS 39180, (601) 636-1605, (800) 862-1300: 17 rms, pb, $75-105; cc-MC, V; c-ltd, s-ltd, d-ltd, p-no, Full Bkfst; h-Glenn Williams. Greek Revival mansion from 1840s features pool and jacuzzi on four acres of grounds.
   Lincoln Ltd. B&B (S), P.O. Box 3479, Meridian, MS 39303, (601) 482-5483.

Roadside food: If you're looking for still more catfish after the event, **Top of the River,** 4150 Washington Street, Vicksburg, (601) 636-6262, serves up nothing but catfish. For a change of pace, southern-cooked vegetables and southern fried chicken are the specialties at **Walnut Hill,** 1214 Adam Street, Vicksburg, (601) 638-4910. "The best steaks in America" are here, say some of the diners at **Doe's Eat Place,** 502 Nelson, Greenville, (601) 334-3315.

Some readings to enhance travels: Brock, Nancy, and Brewer, Nancy, *Traipsin' North Mississippi Roads,* Curtis Media, 1984; Lee, Jasper S., *Commercial Catfish Farming,* Inter Print, 1981; Thigpen, S. G., *Boy in Rural Mississippi,* Thigpen, 1960.

Turn off here along the way: Belzoni lies in the heart of Humphreys County, off the main routes of I-20, I-55, U.S. 61, and U.S. 82. The closest town is called **Hard Cash.** That name accurately reflects the lot of many from the region.

The Delta area is best known for two exports—cotton and the blues. The region around **Greenwood** is known as the largest producer of cotton in America. Over at **Greenville,** the Delta Blues Festival, in September, is the highlight of the years (see page 78). But the music can still be heard not far from U.S. 82 and 61.

If you want to wander and explore, **Jackson,** the state's largest city and its capital, offers attractions that include the **State Capitol** (601) 359-3114 and the **Manship House,** 420 East Fortification Street, (601) 961-4724, a restored Gothic Revival home.

Event: Kentucky Derby Festival
When: Last week in April/First week in May
Where: Louisville, Kentucky

Contact: Kentucky Derby Festival
137 West Muhammad Ali Boulevard
Louisville, KY 40202
(502) 584-6383

Something about the event: This ten-day festival offers more than 70 events, culminating in the running of the Kentucky Derby. Activities include the Pegasus Parade, a hot-air balloon race, steamboat races, square dancing, concerts, and fireworks.

Accommodations with a personal touch:
Log Cabin Bed and Breakfast (B&B), 350 North Broadway, Georgetown, KY 40324, (502) 863-3514: 4 rms (one rental), pb, $56 ($10 each extra person); cc-no; c-yes, s-yes, d-yes, p-yes, Cont Bkfst; h-Janice McKnight. Authentic 1809 log cabin, disassembled and rebuilt at its present site. Old wood and new conveniences combine to provide comfortable accommodations.

Seebach Hotel (H), 500 Fourth Avenue, Louisville, KY 40202, (502) 585-3200: 322 rms, pb, $96-130; cc-AE, DC, MC, V; c-yes, s-ltd, d-yes, p-yes, Bkfst-no. Luxury lives on at this 1905 hotel, with eight murals in lobby and full services.

Kentucky Homes Bed and Breakfast (S), 1431 St. James Court, Louisville, KY 40208, (502) 635-7341.

Roadside food: The **Cracker Barrel,** along I-75, features southern specialties such as cornbread and Kentucky Derby pie (with pecans, chocolate chips, and bourbon). In town, the **Brown Hotel,**

335 West Broadway, (502) 583-1234, serves something called the "hot brown sandwich." It is breast of turkey on toasted points with a mornay sauce and garnished with tomatoes and bacon. They say that the specialty sauce has been used since 1936. **John E's Restaurant and Lounge,** 3708 Bardstown Road, (502) 456-1111, features steak, seafood, ribs, and pork chops.

Some readings to enhance travels: Hood, Fred J., ed., *Kentucky: Its History and Heritage,* Forum Press, 1978; Channing, Steven A., *Kentucky,* Norton, 1977; Federal Writers' Project, American Guide Series, *Kentucky: A Guide to the Bluegrass State,* Hastings, 1954; Courier Journal, *Travels through Kentucky History,* Data Courier, 1976.

Bryant, Beverly, and Williams, Jean, *Portraits in Roses: One Hundred Nine Years of Kentucky Derby Winners,* McGraw-Hill, 1984; Burt, William, *Churchill Downs Museum Book,* Harmony House, 1986; Strode, William, *The Complete Guide to Kentucky Horse Country,* Classic, 1980.

Turn off here along the way: Even if you don't bet on horses, a visit to **Churchill Downs,** 700 Central Avenue in Louisville, will let you get a feel for the city and for the importance it attaches to horses and the Derby. In addition to the track itself, the Downs is home to the **Kentucky Derby Museum,** 700 Central Avenue. It chronicles the history of the race using computerized participatory exhibits and a 360-degree multi-image show.

For the general history of Louisville and Kentucky, see the **Louisville Museum of History and Science,** 727 West Main Street, (502) 589-4584. For the same thing on film, take in the **Kentucky Show at Theatre Square,** (502) 585-4008.

Louisville's **Kentucky Center for the Arts,** 5 Riverfront Plaza, (502) 584-7777, presents opera, orchestra, ballet, and stage performances.

The **Colonel Harland Sanders Museum** at Kentucky Fried Chicken Headquarters, 1441 Gardiner Lane, Louisville, (502) 456-8353, chronicles the growth of the business from a small struggling enterprise to a multi-million-dollar operation.

Many people associate Louisville with the Louisville Slugger baseball bat. In fact, it is made across the river in Indiana. At the **Hillerich-Bradsbury Co.,** 1525 Charleston–New Albany Road, New Albany, Indiana, (812) 288-6611, you can see how bats and golf clubs are made. There is also a museum of famous bats.

Event: Jimmie Rodgers Memorial Festival
When: Usually the last week in May
Where: Meridian, Mississippi

Contact: Jimmie Rodgers Memorial Festival
P.O. Box 1928
Meridian, MS 39305
(601) 693-2686

Something about the event: The festival commemorates the life of the legendary blues singer-songwriter and his impact on country music. There are talent shows, a beauty pageant, gospel singing, street dancing, catfish dinners, barbecues, and all-day music. (See "The Music of America," page 65.)

Accommodations with a personal touch:
   Lincoln B&B (S), P.O. Box 3479, Meridian, MS 39303, (601) 482-5483.

Roadside food: Weidmann's Restaurant, 208 22d Avenue, Meridian, (601) 693-1751, has been a Meridian institution since 1870. They serve ham, chicken steak, seafood, and a specialty—peanut butter with rolls.

Some readings to enhance travels: Skates, John R., *Mississippi,* Norton, 1979; Cash, Wilbur J., *The Mind of the South,* Random House, 1960; Federal Writers' Project, American Guide Series, *Mississippi: A Guide to the Magnolia State,* Hastings, 1938; Thorp, Willard, ed., *A Southern Reader,* Knopf, 1955.
   Paris, Mike, and Comber, Chris, *Jimmie the Kid: The Life of Jimmie Rodgers,* Da Capo, 1981; Portfield, Nolan, *Jimmie Rodgers: The Life and Times of America's Blue Yodeler,* University of Illinois Press, 1979; Rodgers, Carrie, *My Husband, Jimmie Rodgers,* Country Music, 1975.

Turn off here along the way: The **Jimmie Rodgers Memorial Museum,** Highland Park, (601) 485-1808, honors the man known as the "Father of Country Music." There is some of the railroad equipment Rodgers sang about, as well as the singer's guitar and sheet music.
   Meridian was a Confederate headquarters during the Civil War. That was before General Sherman and his Union troops arrived and leveled the town. It has since been rebuilt a number of times.

One of the few Civil War structures to survive was the **Merrehope and F. W. Williams House,** 905 31st Avenue, (601) 483-8439, a 20-room antebellum mansion with ruby glass etched in the front door.

A short drive away is a surprising find—the **Laureen Rodgers Museum of Art,** Fifth Avenue, (601) 649-6374, where you can view works by Homer, Whistler, and Sargent.

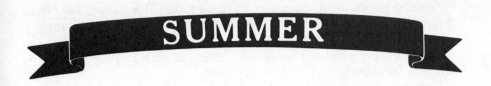

SUMMER

The Music of America

On May 11, 1988, America honored its foremost composer of popular music, Irving Berlin, on the occasion of his 100th birthday. In the process, America ended up celebrating its own rich musical legacy.

On the radio, that day, one could hear the voices of Bing Crosby, Al Jolson, Kate Smith, and of more recent vocalists like Linda Ronstadt and Willie Nelson, all paying homage to Berlin's musical genius. Hearing such music on the airwaves today is becoming more of a rarity as the musical tastes of some change. But it is clear from the musical events around America that Irving Berlin's music and that from the era he represents still remain as popular as ever today.

Those who remember Glenn Miller and his music tend to regard Fort Morgan, Colorado, as the bandleader's home town. But folks in Clarinda, Iowa, see things differently. They regard Glenn Miller as their own because he was born there, even though Matte and Lois Miller moved away when Glenn was four years old. In 1976, during the country's bicentennial celebration, Glenn Miller's first home at 601 South 16th Street in Clarinda was dedicated as a national historic site. What started with a plaque from the local Lion's Club has since grown into an annual Glenn Miller Festival, an event that attracts fans from throughout the United States, as well as from such far-away places as Japan, Germany, and South Africa.

"It's such wonderful music, and it's harder to find on the radio these days," says Wilda Martin of the Glenn Miller Society, which sports a membership of more than six thousand from 40 states and 16 foreign countries. "For at least one weekend, Glenn Miller is again king."

Special guests over the years have included Bob Hope, Jimmy Stewart, who played Miller in *The Glenn Miller Story*, and former members of the Miller Orchestra.

"It's amazing what the sound of the music does to people," says Martin. "Suddenly they feel young again."

Just as invigorating are the sounds of country and western music, a genre that today can be heard as readily in New York City as in Austin, Texas, or Asheville, North Carolina. Jimmie Rodgers, "the Father of Country Music," is credited with having molded diverse musical forms into something new and distinctive.

"Jimmie Rodgers, of course, is a member of the Country Music Hall of Fame," says Jean Bishop of the Jimmie Rodgers Museum in Meridian, Mississippi. "But he is also in the W. C. Handy Blues Hall of Fame and the Rock and Roll Hall of Fame." It was Jimmie Rodgers, she says, who cleared the way for the likes of Elvis Presley and Johnny Cash.

Although Rodgers's career lasted just six years, he sold more than 20 million records. Only the great Caruso sold more. Rodgers's 111 titles include some that were accompanied by jazz greats such as Earl "Fatha" Hines and Louis Armstrong. And although his music is most frequently associated with the railroads, it encompassed much more. "He sang of the whole range of the human experience—family, work, the road," says Jean Bishop. "It was about life."

Each May, Jimmie Rodgers and his music are recalled at the Jimmie Rodgers Memorial Festival in his hometown of Meridian, Mississippi (see page 62). It brings out thousands of fans, along with entertainers like Conway Twitty and Charlie Daniels.

In the 1930s, country music took another evolutionary step with the advent of Tex-Mex music, better known today as western swing. The new sound was created by blending traditional black jazz, country music, and the band sounds coming over the radio from New York and Chicago. It was most popular in the Southwest, and one of the best-known groups was Bob Wills and his Texas Playboys.

Wills started broadcasting on KVVO Radio in Tulsa in 1934. By the late 1930s, he had his own record label and had earned the title "King of Western Swing," a compliment that places him with the likes of Benny Goodman. Wills was one of the first musicians who was equally sensitive to the music of Texas and the music of the eastern cities.

Each May, Wills' fans gather at the annual Bob Wills Festival in his hometown of Turkey, Texas. Wills is no longer around, but former Playboy musicians return each year to please the crowd with such old favorites as "Right or Wrong," "Cowboy Stomp," and "Cherokee Maiden." "It feels like fifty years ago again when they get going," says Laureen Setloff of Turkey.

In the minds of many Americans, the home of American music is New Orleans, made famous by jazz musicians like King Oliver, Jelly Roll Morton, and Louis Armstrong. In the 1970s, when New Orleans jazz was in danger of being lost, a festival was created to showcase the city's rich musical heritage and its modern-day talent. Today, the New Orleans Jazz and Heritage Festival is a major event, drawing three hundred thousand listeners. Continuous music is offered over a ten-day period at various locations around town. There are arts and crafts and traditional Cajun foods such as gumbo, jambalaya, and po' boy sandwiches.

Musically, the festival concentrates on traditional jazz. At the same time, there is a wide range of artists, Pete Fountain and Wynton Marsalis to Fats Domino and Zydeco king Clifton Chenier.

One of the traditional musicians at the festival is Percy Humphrey. A member of the famous Preservation Hall Jazz Band, Percy was born in 1905. Asked how long he has been playing, he answers, "Too long to remember."

"For a long time I thought the music was gonna die. We was playin' just to old folks," he says. "But now it's got new life and young ones, they listen too."

Even in his mid-80s, Humphrey still plays at least twice weekly and travels extensively. "But I've slowed up some lately," he concedes. "You got to."

Does he expect the music to continue?

"Don't know about later, but as long as I'm around, I'll make sure it's played."

It's a sentiment shared by many fans of American music. Blues, bluegrass, or big band, it continues to bond us.

Event: Mountain Dance and Folk Festival
When: First Thursday, Friday and Saturday of August
Where: Asheville, North Carolina

Contact: Festival Manager
Asheville Area Chamber of Commerce
P.O. Box 1011
Asheville, NC 28802
(704) 258-3916

Something about the event: Asheville has hosted this event for more than 60 years. Activities include traditional mountain-style clog and figure dancing, old-time and bluegrass string bands, ballad singing, dulcimer playing, buck dancing, storytelling, and dance and band competitions.

Accommodations with a personal touch:
Albemarle Inn (I), 86 Edgemont Road, Asheville, NC 28801, (704) 255-0027: 20 rms, pb, $50-69; cc-AE, MC, V; c-over 14, s-ltd, d-no, p-no, Full Bkfst; h-John and Rose Mellin. Inn, listed on National Register of Historic Places, situated on one acre. Antiques, off-street parking, and modern conveniences in old-time ambience.

Baird House Country Inn (I), 121 South Main Street, P.O. Box 490, Mars Hill, NC 28754, (704) 689-5722: 5 rms, 2 pb, $40-50; cc-AE; c-yes, s-yes, d-no, p-no, Full Bkfst; h-Yvette Wessel. Inn dates from 1905. Antiques, oriental rugs, and fireplaces in rooms.

Cedar Crest Victorian Inn (I), 674 Biltmore Avenue, Asheville, NC 28803, (704) 252-1389: 10 rms, 8 pb, $60-90; cc-AE, DISC, MC, V; c-over 12, s-ltd, d-ltd, p-no, Cont-Plus Bkfst; h-Barbara and Jack McKewen. Unique Victorian inn with woodwork in each room and a veranda where afternoon tea is served.

Flint Street Inn (I), 116 Flint Street, Asheville, NC 28801, (704) 253-6773: 8 rms, pb, $65; cc-AE, DISC, MC, V; c-over 12, s-yes, d-no, p-no, Full Bkfst; h-Rick and Lynn Vogel. Turn-of-the-century inn in historic district features antiques and collectibles.

Old Reynolds Mansion (I), 100 Reynolds Heights, Asheville, NC 28804, (704) 254-0496: 10 rms, 7 pb, $40-65; cc-no; c-over 5, s-yes, d-no, p-no, Cont Bkfst; h-Fred and Helen Faber. Antebellum home, from 1847, set on four acres of secluded land. Two wrap-around verandas and a swimming pool.

Roadside food: Bill Stanley's BBQ, 20 South Spruce, Asheville, (704) 253-4871, is a local institution. It was featured on Charles Kuralt's television show. You do not come here just to eat, but to take in the bluegrass music and clog dancing. The dancers have traveled the world and have even performed for the Queen of England. **Weaverville Milling Company,** Reems Creek Road, Weaverville, (704) 645-7400, is a converted mill that specializes in local mountain trout and homemade desserts, including handmade ice cream, peanut butter pie, and fresh peach shortcake.

Some readings to enhance travels: Corey, Faris, *Exploring the Mountains of North Carolina,* Provincial, 1987; Costenbader, Carol W., *Insider's Guide to Asheville and Western North Carolina,* Aerial Photo, 1987; Langley, Joan, and Langley, Wright, *Yesterday's Asheville,* Seaman, 1975; Ready, Milton, *Asheville: Lands of the Sky,* Windsor, 1986.

Turn off here along the way: Asheville, a city of 60,000 in western North Carolina, is nestled between the **Great Smokies** and the **Blue Ridge Mountains** at the convergence of the French Broad and Swananoa rivers. Because of its location, it has long been a regional center of commerce and transportation.

The city has maintained many of its old buildings and has preserved its regional mountain music and culture. Weaving, pottery, and silversmithing are prominent. On Saturday nights throughout the summer, mountain folk come into town to perform at what has become known as the **Shindig on the Green**, Town Green at College Street.

One Asheville attraction is the **Biltmore Estate** on U.S. 25, (704) 274-1776, built at the end of the 19th century by the famous Vanderbilts. The estate includes a 250-room chateau filled with art, antiques, even a bowling alley. The estate is also home to a winery and to gardens laid out by Frederick Law Olmsted, the planner of New York's Central Park.

Just east of Asheville is the **Blue Ridge Parkway,** a 470-mile road connecting the **Great Smoky National Park** in the south with the **Shenandoah National Park** in the north. It reaches altitudes as high as 6,000 feet and offers spectacular views. Along the way is the **Folk Art Center** at Milepost 382, (704) 298-7928, which features the crafts, music, and culture of the Southern Highlands.

Event: Hillbilly Day
When: July 4
Where: Mountain Rest, South Carolina

Contact: Hillbilly Day
P.O. Box 34
Mountain Rest, SC 27108
(803) 638-2038

Something about the event: This celebration of traditional crafts and mountain music is held on Independence Day at the Mountain Rest Community Club. There is bluegrass, clogging, and square dancing.

Accommodations with a personal touch:
   The **Old Edwards Inn** (I), Main Street, P.O. Box 1778, Highlands, NC 28741, (704) 526-5036: 21 rms, pb, $65-75; cc-no, AE, MC, V; c-ltd, s-yes, d-no, p-no, Cont Bkfst; h-Jay. 110-year-old restored.
   Duttonwood Inn (I), 190 Georgia Road, Franklin, NC 28734, (704) 369-8985: 5 rms, 3 pb, $45-55; cc-no; c-over 10, s-yes, d-no, p-no, Full Bkfst; h-Liz Oehser. Located opposite recreational area.
   Summit Inn (I), P.O. Box 511, Franklin, NC 28734, (704) 524-2006: 14 rms, 7 pb, $35-40; cc-no; c-yes, s-yes, d-no, p-no, Bkfst-no. Farm, built in 1898, converted to antique-filled inn high in the hills.

Roadside food: Mountain trout, the specialty of the region, is featured on the menu along with North Carolina quail at **The Verandah,** Lake Sequoyah, Highway 64, Highlands, (704) 526-2338. The restaurant has received awards for its wine list. At **Highlands,** Highway 64, (704) 526-4799, the specialty is a seafood platter. Also in Highlands is the **Smoke House BBQ,** Route 64, (704) 652-6414.

Some readings to enhance travels: Roberts, Nancy and Bruce, *South Carolina Ghosts: From the Mountains to the Coast,* University of South Carolina, 1983; Bledsoe, Jerry, *Just Folks: Visitin' with Carolina People,* Globe Pequot, 1980; Taylor, Rossen H., *Carolina Crossroads: A Study of Rural Life at the End of the Horse and Buggy Era,* Johnson, 1966. (See also "Plantation Days," page 81.)

Turn off here along the way: Mountain Rest is situated in the scenic but little publicized western hills of South Carolina, in the midst of the 360,000-acre **Sumter National Forest,** which offers hiking, camping, and white-water rafting in summer. The movie *Deliverance* was filmed here.

On the way to I-85, you'll pass through **Clemson,** the home of **Clemson University,** (803) 656-4791, which was built on land that was once part of the plantation of Vice President John C. Calhoun. Nearby, off U.S. 76, is **Pendleton,** (803) 646-3782, once a summer resort for the wealthy, now a historic district of homes and plantations.

If you stop at **Cousin's General Store,** Route 28, near Mountain Rest, on a Saturday night, you can still hear old-fashioned, authentic bluegrass music. If the weather is good, they'll play outside, right next to the gas pumps. Good music, simple and pure.

Event: Old-Fashioned Fourth of July
When: July 4
Where: White Springs, Florida

Contact: Stephen Foster State Folk Culture Center
P.O. Box 265
White Springs, FL 32096
(904) 397-2192

Something about the event: July Fourth, America's birthday, is also the birthday of the composer Stephen Foster. Both occasions are celebrated in White Springs. There are games, music, picnics, and concerts. The music is all American, with a special focus on Foster favorites such as "Swanee River" and "My Old Kentucky Home."

Accommodations with a personal touch:
   Susina Plantation Inn (I), Route 3, Box 1010, Thomasville, FL 31792, (912) 377-9644: 8 rms, pb, $100-150; cc-no; c-yes, s-yes, d-yes, p-no, Full Bkfst (also dinner); h-Anne Marie Walker. Antique-filled Greek Revival mansion with pool and fishing.

   The **Kenwood** (I), 38 Marie Street, St. Augustine, FL 32084, (904) 824-2116: 132 rms, pb, $55-75; cc-MC, V; c-over 12, s-ltd, d-ltd, p-no, Cont Bkfst; h-Kerri Ann and Mark Constant. Swimming pool, fenced-in courtyard, sherry, and bicycle for guests.

   Casa de Solana (I), 21 Aviles Street, St. Augustine, FL 32084, (904) 824-3555: 4 rms, pb, $100; cc-AE, MC, V; c-yes, s-ltd, d-ltd, p-no, Full Bkfst; h-McMurray Family. Seventh oldest home in town, listed on the National Register of Historic Places. Features turned down sheets and bicycles for guests.

   Suncoast Accommodations (S), 8690 Gulf Boulevard, St. Petersburg, FL 33706, (813) 360-1753.

Roadside food: St. Augustine is home to some fine restaurants. The town's Spanish origins are recalled in the cuisine at the **Columbia Restaurant,** 98 St. George Street, (904) 824-3341. A specialty is snapper à la conte. Local seafood is served at **Salt Water Cowboys,** 299 Dondanville Road, (904) 471-2332, and at **Compton's Seafood Restaurant,** 4100 Coastal Highway, (904) 824-8051, which specializes in fried shrimp.

Some readings to enhance travels: Tebeau, Charlton W., *A History of Florida,* University of Miami Press, 1981; Jahoda, Gloria, *Florida,* Norton, 1976; Federal Writers' Project, American Guide Series, *Florida: A Guide to the Southernmost State,* Norton, 1976.

Foster, Stephen, *Stephen Foster Songbook,* Dover, 1974; Howard, John Tasler, *America's Troubador,* Arden Library, 1982 (reprint of 1943 ed.); Mulligan, H. V., *Stephen Collins Foster,* Gordon Press; Whittlesey, W. R., and Sonneck, O. G., *Catalogue of First Editions of Stephen C. Foster,* Da Capo, 1971 (reprint of 1915 ed.).

Turn off here along the way: The **Stephen Foster State Folk Culture Center** is located on U.S. 41, White Springs, (904) 397-2192. If you're wondering why it happens to be here, just look at a map. You'll see that the river flowing by is the famous Swanee River made famous by Foster in "Old Folks at Home." The Center chronicles Foster's life and music.

The Foster Center is located near the intersection of I-10 and I-75. To the east lies the Atlantic coast, **Jacksonville,** and **St. Augustine,** where Ponce de Leon searched for the Fountain of Youth. To the west lie Tallahassee, the capital city, and the Florida panhandle.

Few people think of Florida as the site of Civil War battles. In fact, a major Confederate victory was achieved here in 1864. There is a museum at the battleground on U.S. 90, (904) 752-3866.

Event: Hemingway Days
When: Third week in July
Where: Key West, Florida

Contact: Hemingway Days Festival
P.O. Box 4045
Key West, FL 33041
(305) 294-4440

Something about the event: This festival in honor of the novelist Ernest Hemingway, who lived in Key West, includes a billfish tournament, a 1930s party at the Hemingway House, arm-wrestling contests, a storytelling competition, journalism awards, and the Hemingway Lookalike Contest.

Accommodations with a personal touch:
B&B on the Ocean (B&B), P.O. Box 378, Big Pine Key, FL 33043, (305) 872-2878: 3 rms, 2 pb, $70; cc-no; c-no, s-no, d-no, p-no, Full Bkfst; h-Kathleen Threlkeld. Ocean location with a private beach, hot tub, and jacuzzi.

Hopp Inn Guest House (I), 5 Man-o-War Drive, Marathon, FL 33053, (305) 743-4118: 5 rms, pb, $40-45; cc-V, MC; c-yes, s-yes, d-no, p-no, Cont Bkfst; h-Joan and Joseph Hopp. Waterfront accommodations, with fishing boat on premises.

The Wicker Guest House (B&B), 913 Duval Street, Key West, FL 33040, (305) 296-4275: 12 rms, 2 pb, $35-85; cc-AE, MC, V; c-yes, s-yes, d-no, p-no, Cont Bkfst; h-Mark and Libby Curtis. Inn features sailboat; massage therapy available.

Bed and Breakfast of the Florida Keys, Inc. (S), P.O. Box 316, Winter Park, FL 32790, (305) 628-3233.

Roadside food: The **Quay Restaurant,** 12 Duval Street, Key West, (305) 294-4446, serves local seafood, along with meat and fowl. **Half Shell Raw Bar,** Lands End Village, 231 Market Street, Key West, (305) 294-7496, also serves seafood, including conch chowder, a local specialty. **Emma's,** 1435 Simonton (at the ocean), Key West, (305) 296-5000, claims to have 108 ways of preparing seafood. Nine to eleven different kinds of fresh fish are served daily.

Some readings to enhance travels: Langley, Joan, and Langley, Wright, *Key West: Images of the Past,* Images Key, 1982; Baker, Carlos, *Ernest Hemingway: A Life Story,* Avon, 1980; Fenton, Charles A., *The Apprenticeship of Ernest Hemingway,* Octogon, 1975;

McClendon, James, *Papa: Hemingway in Key West*, Langley, Press;
Sojka, Gregory, *Ernest Hemingway: The Angler as Artist*, Lang,
1985. (See also "Old-Fashioned Fourth of July," page 71.)

Turn off here along the way: Key West, the southern terminus
of U.S. Route 1, occupies an island at the southernmost end of a
200-mile coral archipelago.

In the 1880s, Key West was the largest city in Florida (population
9,890). Scavenging shipwrecks and making cigars were the sources
of its prosperity. Today Key West continues to be characterized by
the same eclecticism it possessed when it was a meeting place for
people from throughout the Caribbean, though its trade route with
Cuba has been closed.

Sites in town include the **City Cemetery** on Margaret Street,
which holds the remains of the American sailors who died in the
Spanish attack on the U.S.S. Maine in Havana harbor—an attack
that prompted the Spanish-American War.

Key West's historical tie to the sea is on display at the **Lighthouse
Military Museum,** Whitehead Street, (305) 294-0012. The museum
is housed in a former lighthouse keeper's cabin and contains a
lighthouse assembly. The lighthouse itself, built in 1847, offers
scenic views of the sea.

Shipwreck scavenging is the theme of the **Wrecker's Museum,**
372 Duval Street, (305) 794-9502, located in the oldest house in
Key West.

Not to be overlooked is the **Hemingway Home and Museum,**
Whitehead Street, (305) 294-1575, one of the writer's homes and
the place where he wrote *A Farewell to Arms* and *For Whom the
Bell Tolls.*

When you're through with touring, take a moment to gaze at
the beautiful sunset for which Key West is famous.

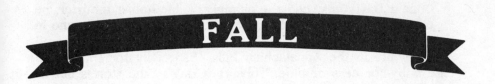

FALL

The Tellers of Short Stories and Long Tales

Before there were radio, television, and the movies, even before there were books, there was storytelling. For years this ancient form of entertainment had been in decline, another victim of the electronic age. But today storytelling is back.

Some form of storytelling is found in every culture around the world. Folk tales, religious legends, bardic myths, and campfire lore are just a few of the many varieties of stories that people tell one another. In America, storytellers can be found in mountain towns and on city streets, in immigrant communities and in old-money enclaves, and their stories may be newly invented or ones that have been told for generations.

For a time, it appeared that the chain of storytelling would be broken by the popularity of television. In the 1970s, a number of groups around the country recognized the threat and set out to revive storytelling as an art.

In Jonesborough, Tennessee, Mayor Jimmy Neil Smith, though not a storyteller himself, was the primary force in getting storytelling going again. He helped start the National Storytelling Festival in 1973, along with the National Association for the Preservation and Perpetuation of Storytelling (NAPPS).

"We realized that we were losing our connection to the genuine, the one-on-one communication of the old tale," says Smith. "For the first festival, we pulled an old wagon into the Courthouse Square and under a warm November sun we told stories."

Today NAPPS is a nationwide organization whose efforts have helped spearhead a rejuvenation of the art of storytelling. These days, though, stories may be shared in a library or a university lecture, instead of on the front porch.

Donald Davis has seen the changes. A Methodist minister, he was introduced to storytelling by his father, a gentleman who in his 80s still tells stories. The younger Davis tells family tales and tales of life in the Appalachian hills. "Especially for those who are baby-boomers or older," observes Davis, "the stories act as a reminder of a rural past, whether it be their own or one they visited. The stories are the museum of our lives. They enable us to look back or touch the familiar too unrecognizable in a contemporary world."

Other localities have also sponsored programs to keep storytelling alive. St. Louis hosts an annual storytelling event at Gateway National Park. And in Kentucky, the Corn Island Storytellers have developed a reputation of their own.

Corn Island's storytelling festival was started in 1976, when twelve storytellers spoke to an audience of nine. In recent years, the festival has drawn over ten thousand people.

As in Jonesborough, the storytellers and their messages vary. One spins an Appalachian legend, the next a Japanese fantasy, the third an autobiographical tale. Ghost stories are told in a cemetery, and there is a storytelling cruise on a riverboat. Of special note are the centenarians, storytellers who have passed their hundredth birthday and are still telling tales.

Frank Smith is a centenarian storyteller. He says he was born to a slave mother in 1867. He started work as a railroad water boy at age 18, served in the Spanish-American War, worked as a bodyguard for Theodore Roosevelt on safari, and traveled the world. His stories recall dog fights, a runaway horse, a groundhog "that tored my boots all to pieces," and a pair of boots that filled with water and nearly got him drowned. "I'm just telling people what I seen," he says. "They're facts about my life, not stories."

Although the American storytelling tradition is most frequently associated with rural folk such as Frank Smith, storytelling has always been a vibrant force in the urban environment as well. One such city storyteller is Penninah Schram, the author of *Jewish Stories One Generation Tells Another*, who lives in Manhattan. Many of her stories concern family and community. "People as they came to North America brought with them their tales, and America became a melting pot of stories," she says.

The apparent differences between urban and rural tales, Schram believes, are superficial. "They're human stories first," she says. "They're basically the same story. It's only the details that differ."

The role of storytelling in an age of electronic entertainment is best summed up in a Native American tale told by Penninah Schram. When television first came to the reservation, the traditional Indian storyteller (the *griot*) found himself without an audience as members of the tribe abandoned him for their new TV sets. But before long, they returned. When the storyteller asked why, he was told: "The television has more than the *griot*, but the *griot* knows me and can help me know myself."

Event: National Storytelling Festival
When: Second weekend in October
Where: Jonesborough, Tennessee

Contact: National Association for the Preservation and
Perpetuation of Storytelling
P.O. Box 112
Jonesborough, TN 37659
(615) 753-2171

Something about the event: This was the first and is now the major storytelling event in the country. Throughout the weekend, there is nonstop storytelling in several large tents. Stories, ballads, tall tales, and fairy tales are included.

Accommodations with a personal touch:
  Hale Springs Inn (I), 110 West Main Street (Town Square), Rogersville, TN 37857, (615) 272-5171: 10 rms, pb, $35-60; cc-AE, MC, V; c-yes, s-yes, d-no, p-yes, Cont Bkfst; h-Stan Price. Historic inn on the town square, built in 1824, is the oldest continuously operating inn in the state. Three presidents stayed there. Antique-filled rooms, many with fireplaces.
  Big Spring Inn (I), 315 North Main, Greenville, TN 37743, (615) 638-2917: 5 rms, 2 pb, $45-70; cc-AE, MC, V; c-over 12, s-ltd, d-no, p-ltd, Full Bkfst; h-Jeanne Driese. Brick Victorian with leaded windows, porches, and antiques.
  Jonesborough Bed and Breakfast (S), P.O. Box 722, Jonesborough, TN 37659, (615) 753-9233.

Roadside food: In Jonesborough, pheasant, trout, and gourmet food are available at the **Troutdale Dining Room,** 412 Sixth Street, (615) 968-9099. The barbecue served at the **Ridgewood Rest,** R.R. 2, Bluff City, (615) 538-7543, has been written up nationally. The restaurant at the **Hale Springs Inn,** Rogersville, 110 West Main Street, (615) 272-5171, dates back to the early 1800s and features two fireplaces and a porch. Hale Springs Inn serves American and Continental cuisine.

Some readings to enhance travels: Corlew, Robert E., *Tennessee,*
University of Tennessee Press, 1981; Dykeman, Wilma, *Tennessee,*
Norton, 1977; Alderson, William T., *Landmarks of Tennessee History,* University of Tennessee Press; Federal Writers' Project, American Guide Series, *Tennessee: A Guide to the State,* Viking, 1939.

Bauman, Richard, *Verbal Art as Performance,* Waveland Press,
1984; Brenneman, Lucille, and Brenneman, Bren, *Once Upon
a Time: A Storytelling Handbook,* Nelson-Hall, 1983; Ransome,
Arthur, *A History of Storytelling,* Folcroft, 1972 (reprint of 1909
ed.); Zimmerman, Morton G., *Tales of a Teller: An Informal Guide
to a Fine Art,* Appleseeds, 1975.

Turn off here along the way: Jonesborough, founded in 1779, is
the state's oldest town, and served as a county capital before there
was a Tennessee. This region was initially part of North Carolina.
When North Carolina ceded the lands west of the mountains to
the United States in 1784, the citizens decided to create their own
state—the State of Franklin. It was the first state created after the
original 13 but was never recognized by Congress and ceased to
exist in 1788. Franklin's first government met at Jonesborough.
Andrew Jackson was an attorney here.

This little-known chapter of American history can be studied
at the **Jonesborough History Museum** in the Visitors Center, 117
Boone Street, Jonesborough, (615) 753-5961. It can also be educational just to walk through the restored streets of Jonesborough.

Event: Delta Blues Festival
When: Third weekend in September
Where: Greenville, Mississippi

Contact: Delta Blues Project
121 South Harvey Street
Greenville, MS 38701
(601) 335-5323

Something about the event: Top national and local blues artists
perform in the area where the blues were born.

Accommodations with a personal touch: See "Catfish Capital of
the World Festival," page 59.

Roadside food: See "Catfish Capital of the World Festival," page
59.

Some readings to enhance travels: Ferris, William, *Blues from the Delta,* Da Capo, 1984 (reprint of 1979 ed.); Charters, Samuel, *The Legacy of the Blues: Art and Lives of Twelve Great Bluesmen,* Da Capo, 1977; Tilton, Jeff T., *Early Downhome Blues: A Musical and Cultural Analysis,* University of Illinois Press, 1977; Mitchell, Peter, *Blow My Blues Away,* Da Capo, 1983 (reprint of 1971 ed.); Oakley, Giles, *The Devil's Music: A History of the Blues,* Harcourt Brace Jovanovich, 1978. (See also "Jimmie Rodgers Memorial Festival," page 59.)

Turn off here along the way: The blues were born in the **Mississippi River Delta**, where the river, the railroad, and the lives of black people inspired the music that has become known as an art form. The **Delta Blues Museum** is located at 114 Delta Avenue, Clarksdale, (601) 624-4461.

To the east, cotton is king along the Yazoo River at Greenwood. The story of cotton, and of Native American history in Mississippi, is told at the **Cottonland Museum,** U.S. 82 West, (601) 453-0925. Cotton plantations were established on what were previously Indian lands. One such plantation that remains is the **Floorewood River Plantation,** Fort Loring Road, Greenville, (601) 455-3821, where costumed guides describe plantation society. There is also a cotton museum at the site.

The history of southern gentility and southern strife can both be seen at Vicksburg, home to numerous antebellum mansions and other structures. The **Vicksburg National Military Park,** 13201 Clay Street, Vicksburg, (601) 636-0583, was the scene of a 47-day siege during the Civil War. The cemetery and Visitor's Center stand witness to the battle and those who perished there.

Event: World's Championship Duck-Calling Contest
When: Thanksgiving week
Where: Stuttgart, Arkansas

Contact: Chamber of Commerce
P.O. Box 932
Stuttgart, AR 72160
(501) 673-1602

Something about the event: The Duck-Calling Contest is the best known event in the Wings over the Prairie Festival. Other activities include a trap shoot, a duck-gumbo cook-off, arts and crafts, and a sportsmen's dinner.

Accommodations with a personal touch:
    Edwardian Inn (I), 317 Biscoe, Helena, AR 72342, (501) 338-9155:
12 rms, pb, $44-59; cc-AE, MC, V; c-yes, s-yes, d-yes, p-ltd, Cont
Bkfst; h-Martha Heidelberger. Edwardian-period accommodations
with parquet floors and beamed ceilings, by the side of a brook.
    Margland II (I), 703 West Second, Pine Bluff, AR 71601, (501)
536-6000: 6 rms, pb, $80; cc-AE, MC, V; c-yes, s-yes, d-yes, p-no,
Cont Bkfst; h-Tara Reynolds. Victorian inn with spiral staircases,
wicker furniture, brick terrace, and home-made breakfast.
    The **Great Southern Hotel** (H), 127 West Cedar, Brinkley, AR
72021, (501) 734-4955: 4 rms, pb, $36-40; cc-AE, DISC, MC, V; c-ltd,
s-no, d-yes, p-no, Full Bkfst; h-Stanley Prince. Restored railroad
hotel, built in 1915, with antiques, ceiling fans, and claw-footed
tubs. The whole area around the train station is being renovated.

Roadside food: What the lobster is to Maine, the catfish is to
Arkansas. Local fish and homemade pies are part of the good old-
fashioned southern fare offered at **The Jones Cafe,** Highway 65,
Pine Bluff, (501) 534-6678. Catfish and many other fish are served
at **Catch of the Day,** Highway 65 South, Pine Bluff, (501) 536-
4242. Over in Old Helena, **Casque's,** at 101 Missouri Street, (501)
338-3565, serves catfish along with fried chicken and hamburgers.
The place may not be fancy, but the food's solidly good. The **Great
Southern Hotel,** 127 W. Cedar, Brinkley, (501) 734-4955, serves
Della rice, which is grown and milled in Brinkley. In addition, the
hotel menu includes Duck Digarod, Arkansas chicken, and catfish
and crawfish (upon request).

Some readings to enhance travel: Ashmore, Harry S., *Arkansas,*
Norton, 1978; Fletcher, John Gould, *Arkansas as a State and a State
of Mind,* University of North Carolina Press, 1947; Hampel, Bet, *The
Pelican Guide to the Ozarks,* Pelican, 1982.
    Barber, Joel, *Wildfowl Decoys,* Dover; Jordan, James M., and
Alcorn, George T., *The Wildflower's Heritage,* JCP, 1984.

Turn off here along the way: Ducks, rice, and fishing are main-
stays of the **Grand Prairies** region of Arkansas, where Stuttgart is
located. It is the lakes and the rice that draw the ducks to the area
to feed and rest.
    To the east is the **Arkansas Post National Memorial** on S.R. 169,
the first permanent European settlement along the Mississippi.

Event: Plantation Days
When: Second week of November
Where: Charleston, South Carolina

Contact: Middleton Place
Ashley River Road
Charleston, SC 29407
(802) 556-6020

Something about the event: At the historic and beautiful Middleton Plantation, you can see traditional harvest activities of the last century. These include making cider and syrup, dipping candles, dyeing wool, spinning yarn, and milking cows. Music and food complete the scene.

Accommodations with a personal touch:
Battery Carriage House (I), 20 South Battery, Charleston, SC 29401, (803) 723-9881, (800) 845-7638: 10 rms, pb, $96; cc-AE, MC, V; c-yes, s-yes, d-yes, p-yes, Full Bkfst; h-Melinda Cass. Located in the historic residential area, near harbor. Home built in 1845 features reproductions. Carriage house was formerly slave quarters.

Elliot House Inn (I), 78 Queen Street, Charleston, SC 29401, (803) 723-1855, (800) 845-7638: 26 rms, pb, $94-107; cc-AE, MC, V; c-yes, s-yes, d-yes, p-no, Cont Bkfst; h-Sherry Bravam. Situated in historic district. Heated jacuzzi in garden courtyard, canopied beds, and 18th-century plantation ambience.

Planters Inn (I), Market at Meeting, Charleston, SC 29401, (803) 722-2345: 41 rms, pb, $89-160; cc-AE, DC, MC, V; c-yes, s-yes, d-no, p-no, Cont Bkfst. Four-star accommodations in an 1840s structure, originally a dry-goods store.

Two Meeting Street Inn (I), 2 Meeting Street, Charleston, SC 29401, (803) 723-7322: 8 rms, 6 pb, $50-125; cc-no; c-no, s-yes, d-ltd, p-no, Cont Bkfst; h-David Spell. Small private inn in an 1890s building, featuring period pieces, reproductions, and an overlook at a historic park.

Vendue Inn (I), 15 Vendue Street, Charleston, SC 29401, (803) 577-7970: 34 rms, pb, $75-180; cc-AE, MC, V; c-yes, s-yes, d-ltd, p-no, Cont Bkfst; h-Harris Goodman. Each room is decorated differently. Wine and cheese are served in indoor garden. Located in historic district.

Roadside food: Charleston is a city of culture and of outstanding eating. **Henry's,** 54 North Market Street (803) 723-4363, offers she-crab soup, stuffed Atlantic flounder, blackened prime ribs, and a special dessert called "Death by Chocolate." **82 Queen,** 82 Queen Street, (803) 723-7591, features "Low Country Cuisine," such as local seafood, grilled duck, and veal, served up with delicately prepared vegetables. The **Multrie Tavern,** 18 Vendue Range, (803) 723-1862, specializes in game pie, chicken and dumplings, and mint juleps.

Some readings to enhance travels: Roberts, Bruce and Nancy, *The Faces of South Carolina,* Doubleday; Johnson, Elmer D., and Sloan, Kathleen L., *South Carolina: A Documentary Profile of the Palmetto State,* University of South Carolina, 1971; Ravenal, St. Julien, *Charleston: The Place and the People,* Southern Place, 1981; Rosen, Robert N., *A Short History of Charleston,* Lexikos, 1982; Wright, Louis B., *South Carolina,* Norton, 1977.

Land, Aubrey C., ed., *Bases of the Plantation Society,* University of South Carolina Press, 1969; Vals-Denuziere, J., *The Homes of the Planters,* Claitors, 1984; Holley, W., et al., *Plantation South,* Da Capo, 1971 (reprint of 1940 ed.).

Turn off here along the way: Middleton Place, Ashley River Road, Charleston, SC, (802) 556-6020, is the oldest landscaped garden in America (circa 1741). The garden is said to have been built by 100 slaves and to have taken ten years to complete. Flowers and trees are on display throughout the year, together with work by craftspeople and artisans.

In the years between the Revolutionary War and the Civil War, **Charleston** was among the most cultured cities in the New World. Lean times brought by the Civil War changed that for almost a century. But the city's unique spirit has been restored and preserved, and is especially visible each spring, when the Spoleto Festival of the Arts is held here.

The historic district remains a viable residential area. It includes 200 buildings from the 1700s and 1800s. Because property taxes in Charleston were assessed by frontage, the city's houses are deep and narrow, with beautiful secluded gardens. These homes can be seen in the area around the **Battery** and **Church Street.**

The starting point for a visit to historic Charleston is the Visitor's Information Center, 55 Calhoun Street, Charleston, SC 29402, (803) 722-8338.

The rice and indigo plantations along Routes 52 and 61 helped bring economic wealth to the area. In addition to Middleton Place, other impressive gardens and former plantations open to the public include **Cypress Gardens,** U.S. 52, 20 miles north of Charleston,

(803) 553-0515; **Drayton Hall,** S.R. 61, southwest of Charleston, (803) 766-0188; **Magnolia Plantation and Gardens,** Ashley River Road (S.R. 61), Charleston, (803) 571-1266; and **Boone Hall Plantation,** U.S. 17, north of Charleston, (803) 884-4371.

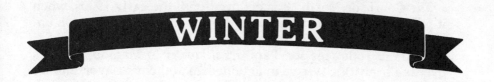

WINTER

The Real Cajun

The 1980s have marked the coming of age of Cajun culture in America. Traditional Cajun dishes like blackened redfish are now found on menus in many city restaurants. There are potato chips with "Cajun spices." Cajun chefs have become celebrities. But Cajun culture in Louisiana goes much deeper than mere culinary delights.

The Cajuns are a community of Francophones far removed from their origins. In 1755, when French Canada fell to the British, six thousand people were deported from the province of Acadia (now Nova Scotia) after refusing to swear allegiance to the Crown. They were dispersed among the colonies and as part of the Treaty of Paris were allowed to relocate to the French territory of Louisiana.

The Acadians shunned the city of New Orleans and settled instead in the bayou country to the south and west, where they encountered French-speaking Creole people from the Caribbean. The Cajuns (the name was shortened from Acadians) have now been living in Louisiana for two hundred years.

Although Paul Prudhomme's restaurant and the Mardi Gras are the best known icons of Cajun culture in New Orleans, the real thing may be seen in the smaller, more traditional celebrations of Mardi Gras (the Tuesday before the beginning of Lent) that are held in places such as Church Point and Mamou. Here the festival is called the Courir de Mardi Gras, the "Fat Tuesday run." Horseback riders cross the countryside, stopping to ask residents for a fat hen or sausage to contribute to the community gumbo that will be served up at day's end, accompanied by fiddle and accordion music. The tradition comes from medieval times, when ceremonial beggars, dressed as jesters, danced in return for donations.

The Courir de Mardi Gras endured until the early 1900s, when it fell victim to modernization and to its own reputation for unbridled rowdiness. It was revived in 1950 by Paul C. Tate, Sr., in Mamou. Today his son Paul, Jr., a lawyer in Mamou, presides over the festivities. "We've maintained an authentic flavor, and it's much more civilized than what goes on in New Orleans," he says.

Horses and riders assemble at 6:30 A.M. in front of the American Legion Home and set out at seven. For the next seven hours, they cruise the countryside, following a route that is kept secret until their departure. In the mid-afternoon the riders make their return to town, where they are greeted with a hero's welcome, and give their collected bounty to the gumbo cooks at the American Legion Hall.

Those preparing the meal, however, do not take any chances. They have plenty of ingredients already on hand. By the day's end, some four thousand people will have tasted their gumbo.

To Paul Tate, the Courir de Mardi Gras and other Cajun celebrations in Mamou go deeper than historic reenactments or party days: "Our culture today survives as a result of much effort of those who take pride in being different. We are first coming to grips with the fact that rather than becoming obsolete as we had once feared, instead our culture is just continuing to evolve to meet the times."

Each June, Mamou also plays host to the Cajun Music Festival, which features traditional music and food, along with such offbeat activities as greased pole-climbing, *boudin* (sausage) eating, and *passe partout* (log cutting). One of the highlights is the Cajun Queen Contest. To be eligible, a contestant must be at least 65 years old. She must also be able to speak French, recite a Cajun recipe, and dance a waltz and two-step.

While Mamou might be an unknown jewel to many English-speaking Americans, it is well known to many French-speaking people from all over the globe.

"Fred's Lounge in town has been written up in all the French-language tour guides," says Tate. "We get folks from France, Belgium, French Canada, and the Ivory Coast, all going out of their way to come to Mamou."

He points with pride to local French culture and especially the French-language classes taught in Grades 4 through 8. It's only one of the community's many ways of ensuring that the language and the culture survive.

"The true basis of our culture is in the way we look at ourselves in our unique politics, our language, and our ethics," says Tate. "For us, Cajun culture is not cool, it is how we live."

Event: A Cajun Christmas
When: December (entire month)
Where: Lafayette, Louisiana

Contact: Lafayette Convention and Visitors Bureau
P.O. Box 52066
Lafayette, LA 70505
(318) 232-3737

Something about the event: There is a month-long calendar of events in Cajun Country to celebrate the season. Homes located on the bayou compete in a yard-decorating contest. Visitors can act as judges on a cruise down Bayou Vermillion. Other activities include exhibits, parades, and concerts. A Living History Christmas Tree is presented by the First Baptist Church at the Cajundome, and there are special open houses, such as the traditional "Christmas on the Teche."

Accommodations with a personal touch:
  Bois des Chenes Plantation (I), 338 North Sterling, Lafayette, LA 70501, (318) 233-7816: 4 rms, pb, $55-100; cc-AE, MC, V; c-yes, s-no, d-yes, p-yes, Full Bkfst; h-Marjorie and Coerte Voorhies. Historic plantation accommodations. Full gourmet Cajun breakfast and chocolate snacks in the evening.
  Ti Frere's House (B&B), 1905 Verot School Road, Lafayette, LA 70508, (318) 984-9347: 3 rms, pb, $45-55; cc-MC, V; c-no, s-ltd, d-no, p-no, Full Bkfst; h-Peggy Mosley. Victorian Cajun home features antique-filled interior, gazebo, plantation breakfasts and evening mint juleps.

Roadside food: If you are looking for real Cajun cooking, the area around Lafayette will not disappoint. By our count, there are twenty eateries that call themselves Cajun or Acadian
  At **Rondol's,** 2320 Kaliste Saloom Road, Lafayette, (318) 981-7080, specialties include steamed crawfish, crabs and blackened redfish. There is music and entertainment nightly and you can tour its seafood processing plant. Another local institution offering Cajun food and song is **Mulate's Cajun Restaurant,** 325 Mills Avenue, Breaux Bridge, (318) 332-4648. Traditional Cajun cuisine is served at breakfast, lunch, and dinner.
  Non-Cajun eateries in the area include **Poor Boy's Riverside Inn,** 240 Tubing Road, Lafayette, (318) 837-4011, which features crawfish and alligator. **Charley G's Seafood Bar and Grill,** 3809

Ambassador Caffery Parkway, Lafayette, (318) 981-0108, offers dishes grilled over southern hardwoods such as mesquite and hickory.

Some readings to enhance travels: Taylor, Joel G., *Louisiana,* Norton, 1976; Rushton, William F., *The Cajuns: From Acadia to Louisiana,* Farrar Straus & Giroux, 1979; Hallowell, Christopher, *People of the Bayou: Cajun Life in Lost America,* Dutton, 1979; Edmunds, Andy, *Let the Good Times Roll: The Complete Cajun Handbook,* Avon, 1984; Federal Writers' Project, American Guide Series, *Louisiana: A State Guide,* rev. ed., Hastings, 1971.

Hornung, Clarence P., *Old-Fashioned Christmas in Illustration,* Dover, 1970; Olliver, Jane, *Doubleday Christmas Treasury,* Doubleday, 1986; Saturday Evening Post Editors, *Saturday Evening Post Christmas Book,* Curtis Publishing, 1976. For books on Christmas crafts, see "Ozark Christmas," page 91.

Turn off here along the way: The Cajuns are descended from French Canadian immigrants, and Lafayette is considered the emotional heart of Cajun Country. In addition to offering food and culture in festivals, this culture and heritage is preserved and studied at the special department of Cajun Cultures at the University of Southwest Louisiana at Lafayette. As a result of its efforts to preserve the French language and culture, Lafayette has become a major cultural city in the French-speaking world, and on occasion hosts Francophone Seminars.

Acadian Village, south of town off of Ridge Road, (318) 981-2364, provides a glimpse of early-19th-century bayou life. Homes, barns, and a chapel have been relocated to the site.

Crowley, to the west along I-10, is called Rice Capital of America. It produces more than a quarter of all the rice in the country and hosts an annual Rice Festival in October.

Event: First Flight Commemoration
When: December 17
Where: Kill Devil Hills, North Carolina

Contact: Visitors' Center
Wright Brothers National Park Service Headquarters
Route 1, Box 675
Manteo, NC 27954
(919) 441-7430

Something about the event: A new world was ushered in by the first powered flight of the Wright Brothers on December 17, 1903, at Kill Devil Hills. On the anniversary of the flight, it is commemorated with a wreath-laying ceremony, speeches, and the induction of new honorees into an air-flight shrine.

Accommodations with a personal touch:
   Ye Old Cherokee Inn (I), 500 Virginia Dare Terrace, Kill Devil Hills, NC 27948, (919) 441-6127: 7 rms, pb, $45-65; cc-AE, MC, V; c-no, s-ltd, d-no, p-no, Cont Bkfst; h-Phyllis and Bob Combs. Beach house 500 feet from beach, within walking distance of Wright monument. Rustic interior. Each room decorated uniquely.
   Crotan Inn Papagayo (I), Route 1, Box 330, Kill Devil Hills, NC 27948, (919) 441-7232: 16 rms, pb, $30-60; cc-MC, V; c-yes, s-yes, d-no, p-no, Cont Bkfst; h-John Link. One mile away from historic site.
   Scarborough Inn (I), U.S. 64 and 264, Box 1310, Manteo, NC 27954, (919) 473-3979: 10 rms, pb, $30-60; cc-DC, MC, V; c-ltd, s-yes, d-yes, p-no, Cont Bkfst; h-Scarborough Family. Recently built structure with old-fashioned look. Whirlpool; antique decorations in rooms.

Roadside food: The Wharf, 12 Mile Post Beach Drive, Naggs Head, (919) 441-7457, features a nightly seafood buffet. At **Darrell's,** Highway 64, Manteo, (919) 473-5366, specialties are grilled tuna and popcorn shrimp.

Some readings to enhance travels: Craig, Barbara, *The Wright Brothers and Their Development of the Airplane,* North Carolina Archives, 1985; Degan, Paula, and Wescott, Lyranne, *Wind and Sand: The Story of the Wright Brothers,* Eastern Acorn, 1983; Howard, Fred, *Wilbur and Orville: A Biography of the Wright Brothers,* Knopf, 1987; Wolko, Howard S., ed., *The Wright Flyer:*

An Engineering Perspective, Smithsonian, 1987. (See also "National Whistler's Convention," page 57.)

Turn off here along the way: The legacy of the Wright Brothers is the theme of the **Wright Brothers National Monument,** Route 158 Bypass, Kill Devil Hills, (919) 441-7430. The Visitors' Center includes full-scale reproductions of the Wrights' glider and flyer machines. There are also replicas of their working and sleeping quarters.

The monument is part of the **Outer Banks,** a 110-mile-stretch of islands and coves along the coast. In late summer and early fall, it is hurricane territory.

Nearby, on **Roanoke Island,** lies the **Fort Raleigh National Historic Site,** off U.S. 641 and 264, (919) 473-5772, where the first English colony in North America was founded in 1585. There are excavations, gardens, and a Visitors' Center chronicling the difficulties encountered by the early English settlers. Roanoke Island was also the site of a major Civil War battle. If you should go, bundle up, for it's cold out there in the winter.

Event: Ozark Christmas
When: First weekend in December
Where: Mountain View, Arkansas

Contact: Ozark Folk Center
Mountain View, AR 72560
(501) 269-3851

Something about the event: Ozark Christmas is a weekend fair with crafts, handmade decorations, food demonstrations and caroling. Evening entertainment features local church groups and school bands and folk music with a Christmas theme. The town of Mountain View is a regional center of Ozark culture.

Accommodations with a personal touch:
   Inn of Mountain View B&B, (I), Route 5, P.O. Box 812, Mountain View, AR 72560, (501) 269-4200: 9 rms, pb, $45-75; cc-AE; c-yes, s-no, d-no, p-no. National Historic Landmark, one block from courthouse square, is said to be the oldest in Arkansas.
   Commercial Hotel on the Square (H), P.O. Box 72, Mountain View, AR 72560, (501) 269-4383: 8 rms, 3 pb, $34-46; cc-AE; c-yes, s-no, d-ltd, p-no, Bkfst-no. Hotel is on the National Register of

Historic Places and dates back to the early 1900s. Wood dressers and iron beds.

Roadside food: The **Ozark Folk Center's** (at Highway 59 and 14 at Folk Center Road, (501) 269-3851, Mountain View) display of Ozark culture stretches into the dining room. Its restaurant serves such traditional items as chicken and dumplings, catfish, ham, beans and turnips, and mountain-style pies. **Grandpa James Dinner Theatre,** Ozark Folk Center Road, Mountain View, (501) 269-3000, serves up good food and a good time. Specialties at the buffet table include ribs, corn bread, beans, mixed greens, and applesauce.

Some readings to enhance travels: Bryant, F. Carlene, *We're All Kin: A Cultural Story of a Mountain Neighborhood,* University of Tennessee Press, 1981; Goehring, Elanor, *Tennessee Folk Culture, An Annotated Bibliography,* University of Tennessee Press, 1982; McWilliams, Dee-Dee, *Yesterday's Lifestyle—Today's Survival: The Life of a Real Ozark Mountain Hillbilly,* Viewpoint Press, 1983; Randolph, Vance, *Ozark Folklore: An Annotated Bibliography,* Vol. 1, University of Missouri Press, 1987. See also "World's Championship Duck-Calling Contest," page 79.)

Hornung, Clarence P., *Old-Fashioned Christmas in Illustration and Decoration,* Dover, 1970; Olliver, Jane, *Doubleday Christmas Treasury,* Doubleday, 1986; *Saturday Evening Post Christmas Book,* Curtis, 1976.

Turn off here along the way: The **Ozark Folk Center,** (501) 769-3851, where the Christmas fair is held, was established to preserve and communicate regional mountain culture, including crafts, music, dance, and the spoken word. Musical programs are scheduled regularly throughout the year.

Event: Confederate Patriots' Birthdays
When: Mid-January
Where: Lexington, Virginia

Contact: Washington and Lee University
Public Information Office
Lexington, VA 24450
(703) 463-8460

Something about the event: The birthdays of two Confederate leaders are observed in Lexington during January. The 19th is the birthday of Gen. Robert E. Lee. The occasion is observed at Washington and Lee University with a convocation. (See "Recalling a Past in Dixie," page 54.) Two days later, the birthday of Gen. Thomas J. "Stonewall" Jackson is marked at his home in Lexington with tours and a party.

Accommodations with a personal touch:
Alexander-Withe (I), 3 West Washington (mail: 11 North Main Street), Lexington, VA 24450, (703) 463-2044: 7 rms, pb, $75 per person ($10 each additional); cc-MC, V; c-yes, s-yes, d-ltd, p-no, Cont-Plus Bkfst. Historic building in town, with antiques and reproductions.

McCampbell House (I), 11 North Main Street, Lexington, VA 24450, (703) 463-2044: 15 rms, pb, $60-80; cc-MC, V; c-yes, s-yes, d-ltd, p-no, Cont-Plus Bkfst. Historic inn located in town.

Maple Hall (I), Route 5 (mail: 11 North Main Street), Lexington, VA 24450: 15 rms, pb, $60-75; cc-MC, V; c-yes, s-yes, d-ltd, p-no, Cont-Plus Bkfst. Country setting on 56 acres. Fishing pond, hiking trails, and, in the summer, tennis and swimming. Restaurant on the premises.

Roadside food: Traditional southern fare is served at the **Virginia House Restaurant,** Route 11, Lexington, (703) 463-3643. Highlights include ham, yams, and biscuits. Fine cuisine using local ingredients may be found at the **Wilson Walker House,** 30 North Main Street, Lexington, (703) 463-3020. But bring your wallet with you. Family-style southern cooking, such as fried chicken, is the fare at the **Southern Inn,** 37 Main Street, Lexington, (703) 463-3612.

Some readings to enhance travels: Dabney, Virginius, *Virginia: The New Dominion,* Doubleday, 1971; Morris, Shirley, *The Pelican Guide to Virginia,* Pelican, 1981; Peters, Margaret T., *A Guidebook to Virginia's Historical Markers,* University Press of Virginia, 1985; Rubin, Louis D., Jr., *Virginia,* Norton, 1977.

Alexander, Holmes, *Washington and Lee,* Western Islands, 1966; Brooks, William E., *Lee of Virginia: A Biography,* Greenwood, 1975 (reprint of 1932 ed.); Connelly, Thomas L., *The Marble Man: Robert E. Lee and His Image in American Society,* Louisiana State University, 1977; Fishwick, Marshall W., *Lee After the War,* Greenwood, 1973 (reprint of 1963 ed.); Flood, Charles B., *Lee: The Last Years,* Houghton Mifflin, 1981.

Turn off here along the way: Located at the intersection of major east–west and north–south routes (now I-81 and I-64), Lexington has always played an important part in the region.

Virginia Military Institute, Institute Boulevard, Lexington, (703) 463-7103, has been in Lexington since 1835, and its graduates have participated in every American war since 1846. One of its most famous instructors was Stonewall Jackson. The **Jackson House,** 8 East Washington Street, (703) 463-2552, and Jackson's burial site on South Main Street, (703) 463-2931, are both located in town. Among its students was George C. Marshall. A museum—at VMI Institute Blvd, Lexington, (703) 463-7103—chronicles Marshall's life and his role as Army Chief of Staff during World War II.

To the north is **Staunton.** First settled in 1732, it is best known as the **birthplace of Woodrow Wilson.** The house in which he was born, a restored Greek Revival mansion, is at Colter and Frederick Streets, (703) 885-0897. Tours of the home and gardens are available. There is also a film.

To the east is the **Blue Ridge Parkway,** a 470-mile thoroughfare connecting Virginia's Shenandoah Mountains in the north to Tennessee's Great Smoky Mountains in the south. The route carries travelers along scenic vistas as high as 6,053 feet. Special caution should be taken if you make the trip during the winter.

MIDWEST

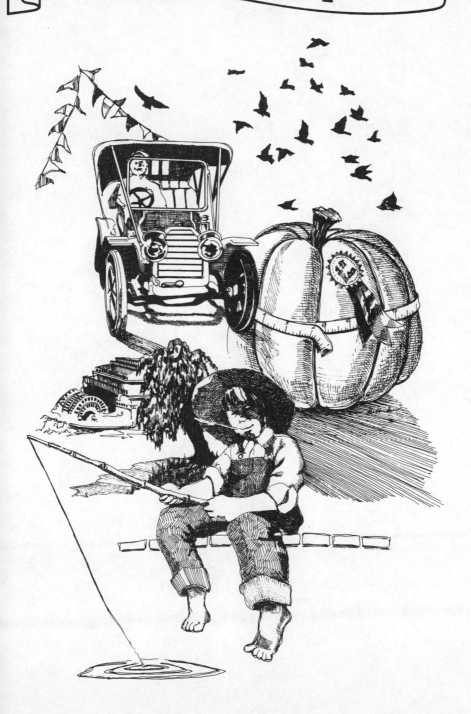

SPRING

Winged Migrations and Other Wonders of Nature

It happens every spring. In fact, it occurs on the same day each spring—March 15. It's one of those inexplicable wonders of nature. But it's not a highly publicized one. The turkey buzzard is not one of the most glamorous creatures, so its return to Hinckley, Ohio, does not garner the same kind of attention as, say, the swallows who return to Capistrano.

The people of Hinckley are not quite sure why the buzzards (also known as turkey vultures) mysteriously return like clockwork every spring. The best explanation is that the buzzards, who live by scavenging, were first attracted to the area by the tons of game carcasses that were left here by hunters in 1818.

No one paid much attention to the buzzards until February 1957, when the *Cleveland Press* printed an article about them. By the time March 15 rolled around, not only did the buzzards return as expected but, surprisingly, there was a large crowd of people there to greet them.

"We didn't know what to do with all the people," says Ruth Moll, who had just moved to town at the time. "In a town of six thousand, we had more than ten thousand who came that day."

Hinckley was overwhelmed. The town's supply of food and drink was cleaned out, motels filled up, and tourist dollars were spent like mad.

Since then, Hinckley has made the return of the buzzards a community event. The town's annual celebration, called Buzzard Sunday (see page 99), takes place on the Sunday nearest to March 15. The Hinckley Chamber of Commerce sponsors games, arts and crafts, and a pancake and sausage breakfast at the elementary school. It also sells buzzard T-shirts, buzzard decals, buzzard patches, and buzzard postcards. The official logo of the Chamber of Commerce is an Al Capp drawing of a turkey buzzard.

The turkey buzzards themselves have not changed their timetable to accommodate the organizers of Buzzard Sunday. They continue faithfully to return to town on March 15, no matter what day of the week it should fall on.

Hinckley's festivities are just one example of the impulse of human beings to marvel at the migration of animal species. Migration is an instinctive behavior that for the most part remains a mystery. At one time it was believed that migration is caused by changes in temperature, but studies have shown that wide variations in climatic conditions have no impact on migratory patterns.

In the United States, the most renowned migration occurs at San Juan Capistrano Mission, near Los Angeles. Huge numbers of swallows have nested at the mission every year since it was built in 1776. They arrive punctually on St. Joseph's Day (March 19) and stay until St. John's Day (October 23) before heading south to Argentina, where they spend the winter.

Not far from Capistrano, in the waters of the Pacific, another migratory wonder occurs: the autumn journey of the grey whales from their northern feeding grounds in the Bering Sea down the coast to Baja California. (See "Mendocino Whale Festival," page 184.) Once hunted almost to extinction—there were only 14 left at the turn of the century—they have flourished under government protection and are now closely observed by scientists and whale enthusiasts. Their migrations are celebrated at the Mendocino–Fort Bragg Whale Festival in March.

Perhaps the most fascinating and touching migration is the return of the salmon to their spawning grounds in the waters of the Pacific Northwest, where they mate and die. As many as 80 percent return to the very spot where they were spawned themselves, some from as far away as six thousand miles.

In Issaquah, Washington, near the spawning grounds at Issaquah Creek, they hold a Salmon Days Festival Each year (see page 208) with parades, kids' events, arts and crafts, and salmon bakes. A sky bridge at the local hatchery allows visitors a view of the salmon swimming upstream, digging nests, and spawning. Tours of the hatchery building are available, but the water is where the action is.

"It's strangely exciting and sad at the same time", says Suzanne Suther of Issaquah. "Especially when the water level is low you can see them jumping and struggling to do what nature says must be done."

People derive a strange satisfaction from watching the migrations. At the mission at Capistrano, Father Paul Martin describes the pleasure he receives from observing migrating swallows and whales.

"It shows me a special mysterious balance," he says. "In a world ever more confusing, it is wonderful to know that certain basic things stay the same without any real explanation as to why."

Event: Buzzard Sunday
When: Sunday nearest March 15
Where: Hinckley, Ohio

Contact: Chamber of Commerce
P.O. Box 354
Hinckley, OH 44233
(216) 237-4242

Something about the event: To celebrate the mysterious return of the turkey buzzards, the residents of Hinckley host games, arts and crafts, and a pancake breakfast.

Accommodations with a personal touch:
Colonial Manor Bed and Breakfast (B&B), 6075 Buffman Road, Seville, OH 44273, (216) 769-3464: 2 rms, pb-no, $30-35; cc-no; c-yes, s-yes, d-no, p-yes, Full Bkfst; h-Jane and Herman Perry. Century-old house remodeled as inn.

Brandywine Falls Inn (I), 8230 Brandywine Road, Northfield, OH 44067, (216) 467-1812: 4 rms (accommodate 12–14), pb and shared bath, $65-95; cc-yes; c-yes; s-yes, d-no, p-ltd, Full Bkfst; h-Katie and George Hoy. A 144-year-old farmhouse located in the Cuyahoga Valley National Recreation area. Inn is leased from the National Park Service. A back barn has also been restored. Parlor rooms, reading room, living room, greenhouse.

Buckeye Bed and Breakfast (S), P.O. Box 130, Powell, OH 43065, (614) 548-4555.

Roadside food: The **Tavern of Richfield,** Route 176 at Route 303, Richfield, (216) 659-3155, prides itself for its Duck à L'orange and an assortment of American cooking. The **Seville Inn,** 39 West Main Street, Seville, (216) 769-3478, features home-cooked meals, Swiss steak, baked chicken, and a salad bar.

Some readings to enhance travels: Collins, William R., *Ohio: The Buckeye State,* 6th ed., Prentice-Hall, 1980; Havighurst, Walter,

Ohio: A Bicentennial History, Norton, 1976; Knepper, George W., *An Ohio Portrait,* Ohio Historical Society, 1976; Roseboom, Eugene H., and Weisenberger, F. P., *A History of Ohio,* 2d ed., Ohio Historical Society, 1977.

Rich, P.V., *New World Vultures with Old World Affinities,* Karger, 1979; Wilbur, Sanford, and Jackson, Jerome, *Vulture Biology and Management,* University of California Press, 1983; Cruckshank, Allan and Helen, *1001 Questions Answered About Birds,* Dodd Mead, 1965; Burton, Robert, *Bird Behavior,* Knopf, 1985; Mead, Chris, *Bird Migration,* Facts on File, 1983.

Turn off here along the way: Hinckley lies halfway between Cleveland and Akron, just off I-70.

Nearby **Bath** is home to the **Hale Farm and Village,** 2686 Oak Hill Drive, Bath, (216) 575-9137. It's a working farm and restored village that offers a glimpse of life in the 1820s. Artisans display period crafts. Special events feature the music and food of the era.

March is still basketball season in Ohio. The Cavaliers play at the **Coliseum,** I-271 and S.R. 303, in Richfield, (216) 659-9100. The Coliseum is part of the development that has occurred along the interstate routes between Ohio's northern cities. At the same time, steps have been taken to preserve some of the area's land from development.

The **Cuyahoga Valley National Park** covers 22 miles of the Cuyahoga Valley between Cleveland and Akron where the Ohio and Erie Canal used to be. Bicyclists, joggers, and hikers now use the routes that were once dominated by commerce. Information is available in the town of Valley View, call (216) 524-1497.

Event: Tulip Time
When: The Wednesday through
Sunday after Mother's Day
Where: Holland, Michigan

Contact: Tulip Time Festival, Inc.
Civic Center
150 West Eighth Street
Holland, MI 49423
(616) 396-4221

Something about the event: They say that there are eight miles of tulips on display at Tulip Time, as the citizens of Holland celebrate the town's Dutch origins. Attractions include Windmill Island, Dutch Village, wooden shoes, street scrubbing, parades, and Dutch music.

Accommodations with a personal touch:
  Wickwood Inn (I), 510 Butler Street, Saugatuck, MI 49453, (616) 857-1097: 11 rms, pb, $80-115; cc-AE, MC, V; c-no, s-yes, d-ltd, p-no, Cont Bkfst (Sunday brunch); h-Dottie. Inn, described as having "comfort and elegance," was selected as one of the nation's top ten inns by *Bride's Magazine.* Located 20 miles from Holland.
  Twin Gables (I), East Lake Street, P.O. Box 881, Saugatuck, MI 49453, (616) 857-4346: 14 rms, pb, $49-84; cc-MC, V; c-ltd, s-ltd, d-yes, p-no, Cont Bkfst; h-Mike and Denise Simcik. Quaint inn a short drive from the festival.
  Old Wing Inn (I), 5298 East 147th Street, Holland, MI 49423, (616) 392-7362: 5 rms, pb-no, $40-55; cc-MC, V; c-yes, s-ltd, d-no, p-no, Cont Bkfst; h-Charles Lorenz. Oldest house in Holland, built 1846, now an antique-filled inn.
  Bed and Breakfast of Grand Rapids (S), 344 College Street, Grand Rapids, MI 49503, (616) 456-7125.

Roadside food: Fresh local lake perch and roast chicken are on the menu at **The Embassy,** 215 Butler Street, Saugatuck, (616) 857-4315. The restaurant sports a classic 1920s interior, including a tile floor. If you're looking for something a bit more elegant, try **Sandpiper,** 2225 South Shore Drive, Macatawa, (616) 335-5866, which offers duckling, seafood, and a superior wine list. A varied menu is offered at **Billy's Boat House,** 449 Water Street, Saugatuck, (313) 857-1188. It ranges from prime ribs to Cajun dishes.

Some readings to enhance travels: Catton, Bruce, *Michigan,* Norton, 1976; Sauter, Richard A., *Michigan: Heart of the Great Lakes,* Kendall-Hunt, 1977.
  Pohl, Kathleen, *Tulips,* Raintree, 1986.

Turn off here along the way: Dutch culture is on display in Holland at the **De Klomp Wooden Shoe and Delft Factory,** U.S. 31N, (616) 399-1803, and at the **Netherlands Museum,** 12th Street and Central Avenue, Holland, (616) 392-9084. The **Poll Museum of Transportation** along U.S. 31, five miles to the north of Holland, (616) 399-1955, includes a large and outstanding collection of antique and classic cars, fire trucks, bicycles, model trains, toy trucks, bottles, and sea shells.

Event: 500 Festival
When: May (entire month)
Where: Indianapolis, Indiana

Contact: 500 Festival Associates
P.O. Box 817
Indianapolis, IN 46206
(317) 636-4556

Something about the event: To stretch out the fun of the famous Indianapolis 500 car race, the city hosts a month-long celebration that includes art exhibits, a parade, children's events, and more.

Accommodations with a personal touch:
  Hollingsworth House Inn (I), 6054 Hollingsworth Road, Indianapolis, IN 46254, (317) 299-6700: 5 rms, pb, $75-120; cc-AE, DC, MC, V; c-over 12, s-ltd, d-yes, p-no, Cont Bkfst. An 1854 Greek Revival farmhouse located on four acres surrounded by undeveloped parkland.
  The **Pairadux Inn** (I), 6363 North Guilford Avenue, Indianapolis, IN 46220, (317) 259-8005: 5 rms, pb, $40-45; cc-MC, V; c-yes, s-yes, d-no, p-no, Cont Bkfst. Located on city's north side, near antique shops, restaurants, and stores.

Roadside food: The food is all-American in this most American of cities. **Hollyhock Hill,** 8110 College Avenue, (317) 251-2294, is a family-style restaurant that features fried chicken, shrimp, and steak. At **Dodd's Steak House,** 5694 North Meridian, (317) 257-1872, they serve steak, fried chicken, homemade pies, and cinnamon croissants.

Some readings to enhance travels: Esary, Logan, *The Indiana Home,* Indiana University Press, 1976; Hoover, Dwight W., *A Pictorial History of Indiana,* Indiana University Press, 1981; Federal Writers' Project, American Guide Series, *Indiana: A Guide to the Hoosier State,* Hastings, 1938; Peckham, Howard H., *Indiana,* Norton, 1976.
  Carnegie, Tom, *Indy Five Hundred: More Than a Race,* McGraw-Hill, 1987; Dorson, Ron, *The Indy Five Hundred,* Norton, 1974; Fox, Jack, *Illustrated History of the Five Hundred,* Hurgness, 1985; Salisbury, David E., et al., *Indianapolis Edition,* Indiana, 1987.

Turn off here along the way: Indianapolis comes as a pleasant surprise to many who know it only from the car race. It is one of America's cleanest and most liveable cities. Founded in 1821, it was laid out on a radial plan, of which the center is the **Soldiers' and Sailors' Monument.**

Restoration has been a major project in town. The cornerstone of these efforts is **Union Station,** the former railroad terminal, which now has stores, restaurants, a movie theater, and a hotel that offers 13 Pullman cars as suites. Union Station lies in the Wholesale District, an area of commercial buildings dating from the last century. Nearby Lockerbie Square features restored homes with cobblestone streets and period streetlights.

As urban awareness blossomed in Indianapolis, so did the city's interest in the arts. The most visible example is the **Circle Theater,** (317) 639-4300, a renovated theater along Monument Circle. It is home to the **Indianapolis Symphony,** among other groups. Indianapolis also has opera, ballet, repertory theater, and jazz.

A visit to the **State Capitol** and the nearby **State Library** can provide a good introduction to the surprising diversity of the state. Another landmark is the **Hoosier Dome,** a 60,000-seat, $80 million indoor stadium that houses the Indianapolis (formerly Baltimore) Colts.

Event: Lewis and Clark Rendezvous
When: Third weekend in May
Where: St. Charles, Missouri

Contact: Tourism Department
P.O. Box 745
St. Charles, MO 63302
(314) 946-7776

Something about the event: The rendezvous is a reenactment of the five-day encampment of Meriwether Lewis and William Clark in 1804 prior to their departure from St. Charles on their epic journey to explore the frontier.

Accommodations with a personal touch:
   Schewegmann House (B&B), 438 West Front, Washington, MO 63090, (314) 239-5025: 9 rms, 7 pb, $35-60; cc-MC, V; c-yes, s-yes, d-yes, p-no, Cont Bkfst; h-George Bocklage. Pre–Civil War inn overlooking the Missouri River features a sitting room and piano. Each room decorated differently.
   Bed and Breakfast of St. Louis, River Country of Missouri and Illinois (S), 1 Grandview Heights, St. Louis, MO 63131, (314) 965-4328.

St. Louis Bed and Breakfast (S), 16 Green Acres Street, St. Louis, MO 63137, (314) 868-2335.

Roadside food: The food is all-American in and around St. Charles. Meat, chicken, and fish are available at **Lewis and Clark's Restaurant and Public House,** 217 South Main Street, St. Charles, (314) 947-3334. Also on Main Street is **C. Broadwaters Restaurant and Seafood Co.,** 920 South Main Street, (314) 946-1111, which features steaks and seafood. At **Williker's,** 1556 County Club Place, (314) 947-1441, the menu ranges from burgers to frogs' legs.

Some readings to enhance travels: Federal Writers' Project, American Guide Series, *Missouri: A Guide to the "Show Me" State,* rev ed., Hastings, 1954; Nagel, Paul C., *Missouri,* Norton, 1977.

De Voto, Bernard, ed., *The Journals of Lewis and Clark,* Houghton, 1953; Satlerfield, Archie, *The Lewis and Clark Trail,* Stackpole, 1978.

Turn off here along the way: First a community of French Canadians, then of German immigrants, St. Charles dates back to 1769.

The town was the state's first capital. A historic district extends south from the former capitol building, and you can take a horse and carriage ride in town. Before you start out, a stop at the **Department of Tourism** is useful. It may be found in the restored train station on Riverside Drive, (314) 946-7776.

Florissant, settled in the 18th century by a French-speaking population, is host to an annual Flower Festival in May. Period homes may still be seen in town.

St. Charles is not far from St. Louis, a city of history and culture in its own right. Highlights there include the **Gateway Arch,** traditional jazz, and rides down the Mississippi River on classic riverboats such as the **Delta Queen** and the **Mississippi Queen,** (800) 543-1949, and the **President,** (314) 621-4040. The **Anheuser-Busch Brewery,** home of Budweiser Beer, is at 13th and Lynch, (314) 577-2626. Tours are available of the historic bottling plant, brewhouse, and testing room. The tour even takes you to meet the company's famous **Clydesdale Horses** up close and personal at **Grant's Farm,** 10501 Gravois, (314) 843-1700. At the **National Bowling Hall of Fame,** 11 Stadium Plaza (across from Busch Stadium), (314) 231-6340, you will find the story of bowling on display in word, picture, and artifact. You can even bowl a game yourself.

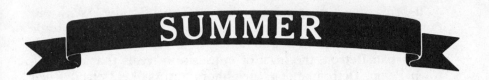

SUMMER

Rally Around the Flag

It's the most American of days. Throughout the land, July Fourth is a day when folks gather to celebrate the nation's birthday. But the day is also a celebration of ourselves and of that diversity that makes us all Americans.

Most often this celebration is to be seen in the small towns of America. There may be a parade on Main Street, a barbecue in the park, or fireworks in the evening sky. It's a scene repeated across the country. (See "Old-Fashioned Fourth of July," page 71.) In the midst of all the parades, hot dogs, and bands, some unique celebrations stand out.

In the Midwest, the "oldest continuous homecoming celebration in America" is held in Pekin, Indiana. (See "Oldest Consecutive Fourth of July Homecoming Celebration," page 107.)

"We've been recognized by the Sons and Daughters of the American Revolution as the oldest," boasts Pekin town historian Marjorie Souder, "and no one has come along to challenge us."

The homecoming started in 1830 and became a tradition, Souder says, when the railroad came to town in the 1840s. Families would meet relatives and friends at the station. Then they'd walk down to the park for a picnic. Over time, this annual walk turned into the traditional July Fourth parade.

Today, the parade includes bands, floats, old cars, and baton twirlers, and is followed by the traditional reading of the Declaration of Independence. It's a day of music, food, and recollections. Trophies are awarded to the youngest person, the oldest, the one attending for the greatest number of consecutive years, and the one who has traveled the farthest to be in Pekin on July Fourth. The town's population, usually a mere nine hundred, swells to ten thousand.

"It brings back people from all over," says Souder. "With our population, it means that rarely do natives get to see the parade because we all have to march in it."

In urban Detroit, the level of enthusiasm rivals that of small-town Pekin. Detroit and its neighbors across the Detroit River in Canada celebrate not only Independence Day but also Canada Day, July 1, which marks the anniversary of the granting of confederation status by the British Crown to the Canadian Dominion in 1867. The cities' International Festival uses these national birthdays to "dramatize the friendship between American and Canadian peoples" along the longest unguarded border in the world.

Conceived by a Detroit journalist, the festival was first held in 1959 and was attended that year by Queen Elizabeth II of England, who was in Canada to mark the opening of the St. Lawrence Seaway.

Today more than one hundred events make up the nation's largest transborder festival. On the American side, the host site is Detroit's University Culture Center, together with the New Center area and downtown Detroit, which offer a variety of musical events, including jazz, Motown, and gospel. On the Canadian side, the Windsor, Ontario, waterfront features music, a carnival, and a casino. Other highlights include boat races, a fireworks display billed as the largest in North America, and a popular international tug-of-war across the river.

There are famous Fourth of July celebrations in major cities, such as the Boston Pops rendition of Sousa's "Stars and Stripes Forever" before hundreds of thousands of fans at the Esplanade along the Charles River, or the Festival of American Folklore on the Mall in Washington, D.C. (see "Independence Day in the Nation's Capital," page 27), or the speeches before the Liberty Bell on Philadelphia's Independence Mall. But there are also some lesser-known celebrations. For instance, in Clay, Kansas, they put on an omelette feed.

Since the early 1980s, employees at the Key Milling Company in Clay Center have awakened early on their day off to whip up omelettes on grills set up on the town square in front of the county courthouse.

Jim Brown of Key Milling explains that twenty-four hundred eggs are broken in advance and the omelette mix is stored in glass jars. When the five-wheel trailer holding the grills is driven into the courthouse square, all that needs to be done is to start them up and cook the eggs.

"We're out there at six," says Brown, "and serving by seven straight through until ten o'clock." Over that time, some twelve hundred people turn out for the breakfast. The price is one dollar apiece, and the proceeds go to the local hospital auxiliary.

Brown warns breakfastgoers to leave their appetites for the town barbecue, which is held after the annual parade. "But it's amazing how much some eat at the breakfast, just to do it all over again at the barbecue a few hours later."

"Rally around the flag" is a popular patriotic theme of the day. In Huntsville, Alabama, they take the saying so seriously that not only do they rally around the flag but into one as well, in the form of a "living flag."

"A few years ago," explains Jo Carr of the Whitesburg Baptist Church, "we got a new minister who was a recent immigrant to America." The minister was so obsessed with being American that he wanted to do something unique. The result was the construction of a 27-foot-by-40-foot "flag" of fifteen hundred lights that holds one hundred singers in its stripes. The flag comes alive for the church's annual pageant, which runs for a week through July Fourth.

"An integration of patriotic music and drama" is how Carr describes it. In the past, musical offerings have included armed forces medleys, Stephen Foster music, and a Civil War story. Representatives of branches of the military present flags of the 50 states.

The highlight of the Huntsville event is the indoor fireworks display. "At first it scared us all," says Carr, "and the fire department did not know what to make of it. But, she adds with a chuckle, "It's still a surprise for the uninitiated when the first fireworks drop from the ceiling."

Event: Oldest Consecutive Fourth of July Homecoming Celebration
When: July 4
Where: Pekin, Indiana

Contact: Homecoming
Route 2, Box 2100
Pekin, IN 47165
(812) 967-4360

Something about the event: This Independence Day celebration is highlighted by a parade, contests for queen, prince, and princess, food, games, and music. The festivities start at 10 A.M..

Accommodations with a personal touch:
Ye Old Scotts Inn (B&B), R.R. 1, Box 1E, Leavenworth, IN 47132, (812) 739-4747: 4 rms, pb-no, $28-30; cc-no, c-no, s-no, d-no, p-no, Cont Bkfst; h-Alliance Ramshaw. Tourist home with veranda overlooks Ohio River.

The **Cliff House** (I), 122 Fairmount Avenue, Madison, IN 47137, (812) 265-5272: 6 rms, pb, $50-70; cc-no; c-yes, s-ltd, d-yes, p-no, Cont Bkfst; h-Joe Breitweiser. Victorian house is more than a century old. Inn features antiques, canopied beds, evening fruits and mints.

Roadside food: Food in the area is described as "good American food," with an emphasis on chicken and steak. The **Plantation House,** South Main Street, Salem, (812) 883-6874, is a family restaurant that features meat loaf for lunch. The fare at **Backroads,** Highway 56 East, Salem, (812) 883-3230, includes steaks and ribs.

Some readings to enhance travels: Giblin, James Cross, *Fireworks, Picnics and Flags,* Clarion, 1983; Schauffer, Robert Haven, *Independence Day, Its Celebration, Spirit and Significance as Related in Prose and Verse,* Dodd, Mead, 1924. See also the readings for "500 Festival," page 102.

Turn off here along the way: The train does not stop in Pekin anymore. You must travel down S.R. 60 to reach the major north–south thoroughfare, I-65. Close to Pekin lies the Ohio River Valley, and across the river is Louisville, Kentucky.

New Albany, situated along the river, was once a major shipbuilding town. The steamship *Robert E. Lee* was built here.

In **Jeffersonville,** also a shipbuilding community, there is a museum that chronicles the history of the steamboat and its importance to the river towns and the country. It's the **Howard Steamboat Museum,** 1101 Market Street, Jeffersonville, (812) 283-3728. Today, Jeffersonville is home to Hillerich and Bradsbury, best known as the maker of **Louisville Slugger** baseball bats. They started in 1859 and also produce hockey sticks and golf clubs. You can see the bats of legendary baseball stars at the museum at **Slugger Park,** 1525 Charleston–New Albany Road, Jeffersonville, (812) 288-6611.

Madison is a 19th-century riverside Victorian community that has been restored to its former splendor. There are old homes such as the Shrewsbury House and Sullivan House. Another highlight is a 1920s downtown area that features antique shops and the beautiful Broadway Fountain.

Event: Lincolnfest
When: Weekend closest to July 4
Where: Springfield, Illinois

Contact: Lincolnfest
P.O. Box 1269
Springfield, IL 62705
(800) 545-7300; (800) 356-7900 (Illinois only)

Something about the event: The historic district of the town where Lincoln practiced law is the location of a two-day celebration that includes a parade, fireworks, nine stages with continuous entertainment, children's booths, musicians, jugglers, and food.

Accommodations with a personal touch:
 Mischler House (B&B), 718 South Eighth Street, Springfield, IL 62703, (217) 523-3714: 2 rms, pb-no, $40; cc-no; c-yes, s-no, d-no, p-ltd, Cont Bkfst; h-Mark and Rhonda Daniels. Century-old house near historic sites and events. Antiques and folk art.
 Hamilton House (I), 500 West Main, Decatur, IL 62522, (217) 429-1669: 5 rms, pb-no, $45-50; cc-AE, MC, V; c-yes, s-yes, d-yes, p-no, Cont Bkfst (also lunch); h-Vickie Schaefer. Homemade muffins are a specialty.

Roadside food: Chili is spelled "chilli" by Springfield natives. A local institution is the **Den Chilli Parlor,** 1216 South Fifth, (217) 522-0123. Another parlor in town uses only one "L" in its name, but the hot stuff is real good there too. It's the **Den Chili Parlor,** 1121 North Grand Avenue East 5000, (217) 544-3000.
 Another specialty to be found in local restaurants is the Horseshoe, an open sandwich with a variety of toppings. Most often it is Welsh rabbit, ham with melted cheese, served with fries alongside. While Horseshoes can be found at almost any restaurant, three eateries that pride themselves on making superior Horseshoes are the **Red Coach Inn,** 301 North Grand Avenue, (217) 522-0198; **Normandy's,** 518 East Capitol, (217) 523-7777; and **Maldaner's,** 222 South Sixth Street, (217) 522-4313. The sandwich is also available in a smaller version called a ponyshoe.

Some readings to enhance travels: Jensen, Richard J., *Illinois*, Norton, 1978; Federal Writers' Project, American Guide Series, *Illinois: A Descriptive and Historical Guide*, 2d ed., Hastings, 1974; Fleming, Thomas, *Living Land of Lincoln*, Readers' Digest Press, 1980.

Russo, Edward J., *Prairie of Promise: Springfield and Sangmor County*, Windsor, 1983; Randall, J. G., *Lincoln, The President from Springfield to Gettysburg*, Peter Smith, 1976.

Turn off here along the way: Of course, the name of Abraham Lincoln is prominent in his hometown. There is a walking tour that guides the visitor through **Lincoln's Springfield.** It includes the National Historic Site—Lincoln's home and burial site, the Visitors Center, the depot from which Lincoln left for Washington, his law offices, the state capitol, and the State Museum. Driving tours are also available.

The **Oliver P. Parks Telephone Museum,** 529 South Seventh Street, (312) 753-8436, exhibits 117 phones of all kinds.

Event: Tom Sawyer Days
When: First week in July
Where: Hannibal, Missouri

Contact: Hannibal Visitors and Convention Bureau
P.O. Box 624
Hannibal, MO 63401
(314) 221-2477

Something about the event: The town where Mark Twain grew up hosts annual events based on his books and stories. Activities include a Fence Painting Contest, a Frog Jumpin' Contest, and Tom Boy and Tom Girl Contests.

Accommodations with a personal touch:

The **Victorian Guest House** (B&B), 3 Stickwell Place, Hannibal, MO 63401, (314) 221-3093: 3 rms, pb-1, $35; cc-no; c-yes, s-yes, d-no, p-yes, Cont Bkfst. Victorian home near the historic area of Hannibal.

Fifth Street Mansion (I), 213 South Fifth Street, Hannibal, MO 63401, (314) 221-0445: 7 rms, 2 pb, $35-55; cc-no; c-yes, s-yes, d-no, p-no, Full Bkfst; h-Donaline and Mike Anriotti. Italianate 1800s mansion features large rooms and location near town.

Bed and Breakfast of St. Louis, River Country of Missouri and Illinois (S), 1 Grandview Heights, St. Louis, MO 63131, (314) 965-4328.

Roadside food: True to Mark Twain's writings, a regional specialty is catfish. It is a feature at **Missouri Territory,** 600 Broadway, Hannibal, (314) 248-1440. The **Bardello,** 111 Bird Street, (314) 221-6111, has a split personality. Downstairs, the food is Cajun; upstairs, where meals are served as part of a bed-and-breakfast inn, it is continental. **Carriage House,** 429 Clinic Road, (314) 248-1313, offers pasta, steak, and crepes as house specialties.

Some readings to enhance travels: Budd, Louis J., *Critical Essays on Mark Twain, 1910-1980,* G. K. Hill, 1983; Rodney, Robert M., ed., *Mark Twain International: A Bibliography and Interpretation of His Worldwide Popularity,* Greenwood, 1982; Spengemann, William C., *Mark Twain and The Backwoods Angel: The Matter of Innocence in the Works of Samuel Clemens,* University of Missouri, (reprint of 1966 ed.). See also "Lewis and Clark Rendezvous," page 103.

Turn off here along the way: The visitor to Hannibal could easily be kept occupied with Twain attractions alone. For example, you can visit the **Mark Twain Caves** on S.R. 79, (314) 221-1666, where Tom and Becky Thatcher were lost in *The Adventures of Tom Sawyer.*

There's the **Mark Twain Boyhood Home and Museum,** Hill Street, Hannibal, (314) 221-9010, a restored home that features period furniture and some Norman Rockwell illustrations of Tom Sawyer. There's also a life-size monument of Tom and Huck Finn on Holiday Hill. Organized tours that can show you Hannibal include **Mark Twain Excursion Boats,** (314) 221-3222, and the **Twainland Express Sightseeing Tours,** (314) 721-5551.

Florida, Missouri, to the west of Hannibal, is Mark Twain's birthplace. The life of the author is on display at the **Mark Twain Birthplace and Museum State Historic Site,** S.R. 107, Mark Twain State Park, (314) 751-3443.

Bethel, also to the west, was settled by Germans in the mid-19th century. Many of its original buildings are still standing and open to the public. The German tradition endures in the form of a local German brass band.

Event: The Great Circus Parade
When: Second weekend in July
Where: Milwaukee, Wisconsin

Contact: Convention and Visitors Bureau
756 North Milwaukee St.
Milwaukee, WI 53202
(414) 273-7222

Something about the event: A traditional circus parade is re-created in an authentic manner, with original antique wooden wagons, animals, marching bands, clowns, and all the other pageantry that used to herald the arrival of the circus in town. Milwaukee is the last stop on the circus train that begins at the Circus World Museum in Baraboo, Wisconsin.

Accommodations with a personal touch:

Washington House Inn (I), West 62 North 573 Washington Avenue, Cedarburg, WI 53102, (414) 375-0208: 12 rms, pb, $55-85; cc-AE, DC, MC, V; c-ltd, s-no, d-ltd, p-no, Cont-Plus Bkfst; h-Liz Brown. Stone building from 1853 is a former stagecoach stop that now includes a pub, a bookstore, a chocolate shop, and two whirlpools.

Stagecoach Inn (I), West 61 North 520 Washington Avenue, Cedarburg, WI 53012, (414) 375-0208: 29 rms, pb, $59-129; cc-AE, DC, MC, V; c-yes, s-yes, d-yes, p-no, Cont Bkfst; h-Judy Drefahl. Victorian inn dates back to mid-1800s.

Phister Hotel (H), 424 East Wisconsin Avenue, Milwaukee, WI 53202, (414) 273-8221: 333 rms, pb, $90-140; cc-AE, DISC, MC, V; c-yes, s-yes, d-yes, p-no, Full Bkfst-ltd. Old elegant hotel restored to former grandeur.

Deorshel's Bed and Breakfast (B&B), North 76116 Lilly Road, Menomonee Falls, WI 53051, (414) 255-7866: 3 rms, pb-no, $35-50; cc-no; c-yes, s-no, d-yes, p-yes, Cont Bkfst; h-Dorothy Waggone. Porched inn sits amid woods.

Hebbring Hotel (H), North 88 West 16697 Appleton Avenue, Menomonee Falls, WI 53051, (414) 273-8222: 10 rms, 2 pb, $29.95-69.95; cc-AE, MC, V; c-yes, s-yes, d-yes, p-no, Cont Bkfst. Victorian hotel from 1892 restored to period.

Bed and Breakfast of Milwaukee (S), 3107 North Dower Avenue, Milwaukee, WI 53211, (414) 342-5030.

Roadside food: The Circus Parade is a Milwaukee tradition. So is German food. **Karl Ratzch's Old World Restaurant,** 320 East

Mason Street, Milwaukee, (414) 276-2720, specializes in schnitzel and sauerbrauten. **Jack Pandl's White Fish Bay Inn,** 1319 East Henry Clay (at 5200 North Lakeshore Boulevard), White Fish Bay, is a 70-year-old restaurant that features German and American food in addition to whitefish. **Three Brothers,** 2414 South St. Clair Street, (414) 481-7530, has Serbian dishes such as game, goat cheese, and burek, a pastry pie. It is housed in what was once a brewery-owned tavern. Just up the street is the **Stone Mill Winery,** North 70 West 6340 Bridge Road, (414) 375-4032, where local wines are served with Wisconsin cheese.

Some readings to enhance travels: Smith, Alice E., *History of Wisconsin,* State Historical Society, 1978; Current, Richard N., *Wisconsin,* Wisconsin House, 1973; Dean, Jill, and Smith, Susan, eds., *Wisconsin: A State for All Seasons,* Wisconsin Tales and Trails, 1972; Federal Writers' Project, American Guide Series, *Wisconsin: A Guide to the Badger State,* rev. ed., Hastings, 1964; Umhoefer, Jim, *All-Season Guide to Wisconsin,* Northwood, 1982; Xan, Erna O., *Wisconsin, My Home,* University of Wisconsin Press, 1975.

    Coxe, Antony D., *A Seat at the Circus,* Shoestring, 1980; Eckley, Wilton, *The American Circus,* G. K. Hall, 1984; Freeman, Larry G., *The Big Top Circus Days,* American Life Foundation–Century House Books, 1974; Parkinson, Tom, and Fox, Charles P., *The Circus Moves by Rail,* Midwest Old Settlers; Speaight, G. *The History of the Circus,* A.S. Barnes, 1980; Yarnall, Agnes, *Circus World: Sculpture and Poetry,* Dorrance, 1982.

Turn off here along the way: Baseball's Brewers alternately make their fans cheer and cry at **County Stadium,** Stadium Expressway, (414) 278-7711. The restaurant at the ballpark is open even when the Brewers are not playing. The food there is known throughout the major leagues for its quality.

    Fishing, swimming, and boating are available at the lakefront. The Rainbow Summer program at the **Performing Arts Center,** on the lakefront, 929 North Water Street, (414) 273-7026, offers noontime and evening performances.

    The home of **Circus World** in Baraboo is the old winter headquarters of the Ringling Brothers Barnum and Bailey Circus, S.R. 113 at 426 Water Street, (608) 356-8341. There you can relive the history of the circus. There are all of the wagons, posters, calliopes, sideshows—even a circus in miniature.

Event: National Hobo Convention
When: First Saturday in August
Where: Britt, Iowa

Contact: Chamber of Commerce
P.O. Box 63
Britt, Iowa 50423
(515) 843-3867

Something about the event: In the Depression, Britt was a transfer point for the destitute people who rode the rails. Before long, it became known as a gathering place for hoboes. After many years, local folks decided not to fight the image and to celebrate its notoriety instead. Today hoboes from across the country gather there each August. Activities include a hobo parade, arts and crafts, and food, especially mulligan stew.

Accommodations with a personal touch:
  Bed and Breakfast in Iowa, Ltd. (S), 7104 Franklin Avenue, Des Moines, IA 50322, (515) 277-9018.

Roadside food: The culinary highlight of the Hobo Convention is a stew prepared by the local Boy Scouts. If you're looking for more traditional eats, try the **We-3 Inn,** 8 Second Street NW, (515) 843-3895, which offers a wide variety of American food. At **Paradise Donuts,** South Main Street, (314) 843-3898, there's more than just homemade donuts. They make their own breads, soups, and sandwiches as well. A recent addition to Britt's culinary scene is **Piccadilly Circus Pizza,** Main Street, (515) 843-4600. It is said to have converted folks from the pizza chains and franchises.

Some readings to enhance travels: Childs, Marquis, and Engel, Paul, *This Is Iowa,* Iowa State University, 1982; Federal Writers' Project, American Guide Series, *Iowa: A Guide to the Heritage State,* Hastings, 1938; Pelton, Beulah, *We Belong to the Land,* Iowa State University, 1984; Sage, Leland L., *A History of Iowa,* Iowa State University Press, 1974; Wall, Joseph F., *Iowa,* Norton, 1978; Zelinski, John, *Unknown Iowa,* Wallace-Homestead, 1975.
  Ribton, Turner C. J., *A History of Vagrants and Vagrancy and Beggars and Beggary,* Patterson Smith, 1972; Stevens, Irving L., *Fishbones: Hoboing in the Nineteen Thirties,* Moosehead Productions, 1983.

Turn off here along the way: Within driving range of Britt lie two places of note.

To the northeast is Forest City, the home of **Winnebago Industries.** At the Visitor Center on U.S. 69, (515) 582-6936, you can catch a film and exhibit about the famous manufacturer of recreational vehicles.

To the east is Mason City, named for its early connection to the Masonic order. Meredith Wilson, a local boy, used Mason City as a model for the town in his musical "The Music Man." It is also home to the **McNider Museum,** 303 Second Street SE, (515) 421-3666, whose collection includes 19th- and 20th-century art and Bill Baird puppets.

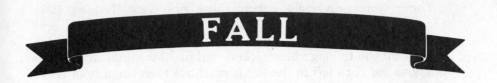

FALL

Champions of Cornhusking

Once it was the only way to get the job done. Then it became popular as a competitive endeavor, drawing crowds in excess of one hundred thousand. For the finals, folks come from across the Midwest. There is no ball, no goal, no track. They simply make a sport of a common job done well.

The National Cornhusking Championship started back in 1924 with a few fast-handed huskers from Iowa, Illinois, and Nebraska. Back then, before mechanization, all husking—removal of the coarse layers that enclose the ear of corn—was done by hand, one stalk at a time. It was one of the more tedious tasks of farm life. Farmers and agricultural historians say that hand-husking occupied more time than any other corn-growing job and was the most costly aspect of the operation.

To make this manual job more efficient and entertaining, a number of techniques were developed that turned cornhusking into something like a sport. Naturally, this gave rise to the idea of holding competitions—first regional, then national. The popularity of these contests reached its peak between the two world wars, when modes of transportation made them more accessible to people across the Farm Belt. Cornhusking champions were treated with the kind of acclaim reserved for Olympians.

The national event was suspended in 1942 because of World War II. The suspension turned out to be more permanent than first thought. Although some farmers kept an acre or so free for practice in hand-husking, most retired their husking hooks and turned to mechanization. Cornhusking contests faded almost completely from the scene until the early 1970s, when the idea was revived at Living History Farms in Des Moines, Iowa. (See "National Cornhusking Championships," page 119.)

There were only eight entrants the first year, but by 1986 the number had grown to 82, with competition offered in several classes (open, novice, ladies, and old timers). Contestants are judged on the tonnage handpicked within 30 minutes, minus deductions for corn left in the fields or shucks left on ears of corn. The good ones can do up to five hundred pounds in that time.

"It's a skill with a lot of work," explains Miriam Dunlap of Living History Farms. "The best of them can keep an ear of corn up in the air at all times."

Unlike many other sports, age is no barrier in husking. "Hand-husking is more an art and skill than a measure of muscle," says the Farm's Vince King. "There are 20- to 25-year-old folks in those contests too. But most of the better huskers are 40 to 60. The good ones have had many years' experience in the hand-husking era."

Tony Polich of Des Moines, Iowa, is one such veteran. A 1983 champion at the age of 71, he was timed at 53 ears per minute and picked 349 pounds in 20 minutes.

"You've just gotta get a hold of the ear and pull," says Polich succinctly.

Polich has been shucking corn as far back as he can recall. He first competed in contests in 1936 and placed in the top 25. He finds that corn has changed over the years.

"In the earlier years it was easier," he says. "Today they breed corn chemically to stay on the stalks more securely, but that makes them harder to shuck."

Asked what his secret is, Polich replies, "It's easy. I learned to do it fast because I had to. Guys today do it for sport. To me it was my life."

Nonetheless, Polich says, certain things can be done to make one a better husker. Most of all, he maintains, practice is essential. "I start a month or so before, to get into practice. You don't forget it—it's like riding a bicycle. But you've got to be careful of getting chapped hands."

"It's all in the hand," says Polich. But, he adds, "Anyone can learn."

Event: National Cornhusking Championship
When: First full weekend in October
Where: Des Moines, Iowa

Contact: Living History Farms
2600 Northwest 111th
Des Moines, IA 50322
(515) 278-5286

Something about the event: Championship meet with competitions in four categories, revived from the years between the world wars. There is food and fiddling as well.

Accommodations with a personal touch:
   Walden Acres (B&B), c/o Briley, R.r. 1, Box 30, Adel, IA 50003, (515) 987-1338: 3 rms, pb-no, $40-50 ($10 per child); cc-no; c-yes, s-ltd, d-no, p-ltd, Full Bkfst; h-Phyllis Briley. Inn, located at edge of Des Moines, is former home of baseball star Bob Feller. Antique shop on premises.
   Heritage House (B&B), c/o A. and I. Vander Wilt, Route 1, Leighton, IA 50143, (515) 626-3092: 2 rms, pb-no, $35; cc-no; c-yes, s-ltd, d-no, p-no, Full Bkfst; h-Iola Vander Wilt. Dairy farm B&B with rooms decorated in Victorian antiques.
   Hotel Brooklyn (I), 154 Front Street, Brooklyn, IA 52211, (515) 522-9229: 7 rms, 2 pb, $16-28; cc-no; c-yes, s-no, d-no, p-no, Bkfst-no; h-Mrs. Kay Lawson. Structure, built in 1875, is on National Register of Historic Homes.
   Bed and Breakfast in Iowa (S), 7104 Franklin Avenue, Des Moines, IA 50322, (515) 277-9018.

Roadside food: At the **Kaplan Hat Company,** 307 Court Avenue, Des Moines, (515) 243-1414, the menu features fettucini, stir-fried vegetables, and steak. An old-world atmosphere prevails at **Bavarian House,** 5220 Northeast 14th, (515) 266-1173. As the name indicates, the food is German. The highlight is a platter that includes sauerbraten, schnitzel, brockwurst, and German potato salad.

Some readings to enhance travels: *Corn: Use for the Whole Corn Recipe and Suggestions Book,* Cookbook Consortium, 1984; Mangelsdorf, Paul C., *Corn: Its Origin, Evolution and Development,* Harvard University Press, 1974; Andrews, Clarence, *Growing Up in the Midwest,* Iowa State University Press, 1981. See also "National Hobo Convention," page 114.

Turn off here along the way: Living History Farms is a museum covering 600 acres. It is dedicated to preserving pioneer skills and the pioneer spirit. The items on display include an Indian village and a variety of working farms that cover a number of periods. There is a general store, a schoolhouse, and other businesses.

In Des Moines, the state capital, you can see the **State Capitol,** East 9th and Grand Avenue (off I-235), (515) 281-5011, with its 275-foot-high dome; the **Historical Museum,** Des Moines, 600 East Locust, (515) 281-5111, the **Art Center,** 4700 Grand Avenue, (515) 277-4405, and **Court Avenue,** Court Avenue, downtown, (515) 286-4950, where restored buildings have been turned into an entertainment area of cafes, restaurants, and clubs.

If you're a train buff, Colfax is a place to stop. At **Trainland,** Highway 117 North, (515) 674-3813, there is a Lionel train display that took five years to build and that shows the development of the transcontinental railroad. Lionel cars dating back to 1911 are on display.

Event: Old Car Festival
When: Second weekend in September
Where: Dearborn, Michigan

Contact: Henry Ford Museum
20900 Oakwood Boulevard
Dearborn, MI 48121
(313) 271-1976

Something about the event: Hundreds of antique vehicles from the turn of the century through 1929 are exhibited at the Henry Ford Museum. Antique car owners bring their restored machines. There are special activities and the museum's regular display. This event is a counterpart to the Motor Muster, held at the museum in August, which features cars of the era between the 1930s and 1950s and music of the period.

Accommodations with a personal touch:
Blanche House Inn (I), 506 Park View Drive, Detroit, MI 48214, (313) 822-7090: 6 rms, pb, $60-70; cc-AE, MC, V; c-yes, s-yes, d-yes, p-ltd, Cont Bkfst; h-Mary Jean Shannon. Inn is a historic site. An antique-filled colonial, located near the Detroit River and close to the mayor's mansion.
Dearborn Inn (I), 20301 Oakwood Boulevard, Dearborn, MI

48124, (313) 271-2700: 237 rms, pb, $95-185; cc-AE, DC, MC, V; c-yes, s-yes, d-yes, p-yes, Bkfst-no. Inn built by Henry Ford, circa 1931, recently renovated.

Barclay Inn (H), 145 North Hunter Boulevard, Birmingham, MI 48001, (313) 646-7300: 128 rms, pb, $72.50-110; cc-AE, DC, DISC, MC, V; c-yes, s-ltd, d-yes, p-no, Cont Bkfst. Hotel features Queen Elizabeth-style antiques and afternoon tea in the lobby.

Betsy Ross Bed and Breakfast (S), 3057 Betsy Ross Drive, Bloomfield Hills, MI 48103, (313) 646-5357.

Roadside food: Topper, 21918 Michigan Avenue, Dearborn, (313) 278-9292, serves lake perch, lamb stew, braised short ribs, and barbecue. **Chamberton's** (at the Holiday Inn), 22900 Michigan Avenue, Dearborn, (313) 278-6900, serves seafood as part of its varied menu. Detroit, not far away, offers a variety of eating opportunities. You can dine on the Detroit River on the **Star of Detroit,** 20 East Atwater Street, Detroit, (313) 259-9160, or get classic Motown food at **Mattie's Barbecue,** 11728 Dexter, (313) 869-6331, where the menu includes ribs, steaks, and chicken and dumplings. Desserts are the specialty at the **Cozy Cafe,** 15 Forest Place, Plymouth, (313) 455-3310. They serve a walnut-raisin sweet roll and some 18 different homemade pies daily.

Some readings to enhance travels: Santer, Richard A., *Michigan: Heart of the Great Lakes,* Kendall-Hunt, 1977; Lacey, Robert, *Ford: The Men and The Machine,* Ballantine, 1987; Berger, Michael L., *The Devil Wagon in God's Country: The Automobile and Social Change in Rural America, Nineteen Three to Nineteen Twenty-Nine,* Shoe String, 1979; Demaus, A. B., *Motoring in the Twenties and Thirties,* David and Charles, 1979; Taylor, William R., *Auto Museum Directory, U.S.A.,* Editorial Review, 1983.

Turn off here along the way: The **Henry Ford Museum** is part of a two-museum complex near Detroit (the other is Greenfield Village) that chronicles the growth of America from a rural to an industrial society. Its permanent exhibit, "The Automobile in American Life," describes the history of American road travel and its impact on society. The museum also covers other aspects of American life, such as home furnishings, communications, and entertainment.

Greenfield Village, 20900 Oakwood Boulevard, Dearborn, (313) 271-1620, is a 240-acre outdoor museum with actual houses and buildings that were moved to the site of the Ford Museum. They reflect the growth of industrialized America.

The museum can keep one occupied for days. But there is more to be seen in Dearborn.

The **Henry Ford Estate,** Fair Lane, Dearborn, (313) 593-5590, is a 56-room National Historic Landmark situated on 72 acres. It includes a self-sufficient powerhouse, underground tunnels, boathouses, nature trails, and gardens.

The **Dearborn Historical Museum,** 21950 Michigan Avenue, (313) 565-3000, chronicles Dearbornville long before Henry Ford.

The **Dearborn Trolley,** 23500 Paril Avenue, (313) 274-6300, provides cheap and entertaining transportation around the town's sites.

Event: Wine and Harvest Festival
When: Third weekend in September
Where: Cedarburg, Wisconsin

Contact: Wine and Harvest Festival
P.O. Box 204
Cedarburg, WI 53102
(414) 377-8020

Something about the event: Grape stomping is the highlight of this harvest event. (Some of the best stompers in past years have been members of the Milwaukee Ballet.) Other activities include arts and crafts, an antiques show, logging competitions, and the making of a giant fish stew. The festival is held at the Cedar Creek Settlement and in downtown Cedarburg.

Accommodations with a personal touch: See "The Great Circus Parade," page 112.

Some readings to enhance travels: Adams, Leon D., *Commonsense Book of Wine*, 4th ed., McGraw-Hill, 1986; Cox, Jeff, *From Vines to Wines: The Complete Step by Step Guide to Growing Grapes in Your Backyard and Making Wine*, Harper & Row, 1985. See also "The Great Circus Parade," page 113.

Turn off here along the way: In the mid-1800s Cedarburg was a vibrant industrial town. Many of its historic buildings and structures have been preserved. The **Brewery Works,** West 62 North 718 Riveredge Drive, (414) 377-7220, and the **Cedar Creek Settlement,** Junction S.R. 57, 143, and County Road I, (414) 377-8020, a former mill, are examples of industrial plants that have been converted to art studios and shops.

Visitors are welcome at **Green Meadows Farm,** a dairy farm west of Waterford on Route 20, (414) 534-2891, and at the **Hoppe Homestead Farms** (an area attraction since 1866), 33701 Hill Valley Drive, East Troy, (414) 534-6480, which offers pony rides and hay to roll in.

The turning leaves of fall can be enjoyed from vintage railroad cars along the line of the **Kettle Moraine Scenic Steam Train,** (414) 966-2866. The train is pulled by a steam engine. Trips depart from the North Lake Depot, Highway 83.

Event: Circleville Pumpkin Show
When: Mid-October
Where: Circleville, Ohio

Contact: Circleville Pumpkin Show
308 Northridge Road
Circleville, OH 43113
(614) 474-4224

Something about the event: Billed as "The Greatest Free Show On Earth," the Circleville Show has been a yearly event since 1903 (except for during WW II). There one can find the world's largest pumpkin pie (350 pounds and five feet in diameter). There are also bands, floats, and all kinds of pumpkin dishes. It attracts 400,000 annually.

Accommodations with a personal touch:
  B&B of Hocking County (S), 15459 S.R. 328, Logan, OH 43138, (614) 385-3935, (800) HOCKING.
  Waynesville Guest Haus (B&B), 117 Main Street, P.O. Box 592, Waynesville, OH 45068, (513) 897-3811: 5 rms, pb, $40-60; cc-no; c-yes, s-yes, d-ltd, p-no, Cont Bkfst. Antique-filled suites, within driving distance of Circleville.

Roadside food: The food is home-style and good in this rural Ohio community. Sausage products are the specialty at **Bob Evans Farm,** U.S. 23, (614) 474-5009. **Hoover's,** 101 Main Street, (614) 474-6623, specializes in gourmet sandwiches. For dessert, you might consider **Tinks,** 2815 Court Street, (614) 474-3065, for a piece of hot fudge ice cream pie. The lunch and dinner menus feature chicken liver.

Some readings to enhance travels: MaCallum, Anne C., *Pumpkin! Lore, History, Outlandish Facts and Good Eating,* Heather Foundation, 1986. See also "Buzzard Sunday," page 99.

Turn off here along the way: Circleville is situated in southern Ohio's farm country, halfway between Columbus and Chillicothe along U.S. 22.

Columbus, the state capital, is nicknamed "Test Market, U.S.A." It was the first place to introduce cable television, interactive television, and home banking. Places to visit in Columbus include the **State Capitol,** Broad and High Streets, (614) 466-2125, a domed Greek Revival structure built in 1861.

The **Columbus Zoo,** 4 miles from town, S.R. 257 at U.S. 33 and S.R. 161, (614) 889-9471, has been highly successful in breeding animals in captivity. There are 100 acres of gardens and exhibits.

Franklin Park Conservatory, 1777 East Broad Street and Nelson Road, Franklin, (614) 222-7447, is a 12,000-square-foot glass structure built in 1859 and modeled after London's famous Crystal Palace. Technology and science are on display at Franklin's **Center of Science and Industry (COSI),** 280 East Broad Street, Franklin, (614) 228-6362.

South of Columbus, on U.S. 22, lies Chillicothe, Ohio's capital in the early 1800s. Many period mansions still stand, including **Apena,** (614) 777-1500, a Georgian mansion dating back to 1906. The history of the area can be studied at the **Ross County Historical Society Museum,** 45 West Fifth Street, (614) 772-1936. It exhibits Indian artifacts and items from the Revolutionary and Civil War periods.

History may also be felt in **Lancaster,** to the northwest of Circleville. The building of canals and railways spurred Lancaster's growth in the last century. The city's past is seen in its architecture, including **Square 13,** near Main and Broad Streets.

To the west of Circleville is **Washington Court House,** which used to be called Washington until the folks there decided they wanted something more distinctive. The courthouse there displays paintings.

Event: National Farm Toy Show
When: Second weekend in November
Where: Dyersville, Iowa

Contact: Toy Farmer
Route 2, Box 5
La Moure, ND 58458
(701) 883-5107

Something about the event: The show exhibits more than 250,000 farm toys produced over the last eight decades, including miniature toy tractors. There are contests and a toy auction.

Accommodations with a personal touch:
   Redstone Inn (H), Fifth and Bluff, Dubuque, IA 52001, (319) 582-1890: 16 rms, pb, $50-140; cc-MC, V; c-yes, s-yes, d-no, p-no, Cont Bkfst. Antique-filled chateau-style inn.
   Stout House (B&B), Fifth and Bluff, Dubuque, IA 52001, (319) 582-1890: 6 rms, pb, $65-80; cc-AE, DC, MC, V; c-yes, s-ltd, d-no, p-no. Victorian inn from 1890.
   Bed and Breakfast in Iowa (S), 7104 Franklin Avenue, Des Moines, IA 50322, (515) 277-9018.

Roadside food: The main foods grown in the area are grain and beef. Beef shows up frequently in Dyersville's restaurants. **Hugo's,** 124 Third Street NE, (319) 875-2167, specializes in prime ribs. **Dick's Steak House,** 226 First Avenue E, (319) 875-7110, serves steak, fish, poultry, and a smorgasbord. **Royal Supper Club,** 703 13th Avenue SE, (319) 875-8410, features steak, prime ribs, catfish, cod, and homemade soup.

Some readings to enhance travels: Harkoner, Helen B., *Farms and Farmers in Art* (for children), Lerner, 1965; Gottschalk, Lillian, *American Toy Cars and Trucks, 1894 to 1942*, Abbeville Press, 1986; O'Brien, Richard, *Collecting Toys*, Applied Arts, 1975; Peake, Pamela, *Making Your Own Toys*, Rodale Press, 1986. See also "National Hobo Convention," page 114.

Turn off here along the way: Twenty-five miles east of Dyersville, on U.S. 20, lies Dubuque, Iowa's oldest town. It was founded in 1788 by a French trader. The primary industries, formerly mining and sawmilling, are now meatpacking and manufacturing.
   On the way into town is a former train line that runs along the Little Maqualea River. Now called **Heritage Trail,** it goes past

old Indian, railroad, and mining sites. Hiking and bicycling are permitted.

Dubuque has a historic district that may be seen by guided or self-guided tour. It also has a unique Egyptian-style jail turned art museum, a railway that offers panoramic views, and stern-wheeler rides on the Mississippi. For information about all these activities, call Dubuque Visitors Information at (319) 557-9200.

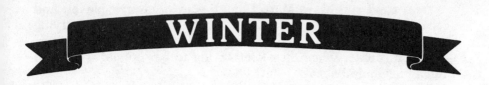

WINTER

Making the Best Out of Winter

It starts in November, slowly at first. It reaches major proportions in December. By January it's in full force—a flood of Americans heading south in search of warmth and sun.

Of course, there are many others who stay behind. Some of them simply grit their teeth and endure the cold. But some actually enjoy it. To these folks, the snow and cold are but a minor inconvenience to be overcome.

In January, for example, you'll find plenty of golfers in Pebble Beach, Palm Springs, and Doral. But you'll find them in Grand Haven, Michigan, as well, at the Polar Ice Cap Golf Tournament (see page 129), where hundreds of golfers ranging from teenagers to retirees brave the elements in 9- and 18-hole competitions on frozen Spring Lake.

"I clear out the lake and create a fairway which is a shoveled-out area the length of a shovel," says Steve Berson, chairman of the tournament, who also acts as greenskeeper—or rather, icekeeper.

Although the course itself is arranged however Berson decides, there are rules to be observed. Only five, seven, and nine irons and a putter are permitted. If the ball is lost, there is a time limit before it must be replaced with a new ball. All balls have streamers attached. For obvious reasons, orange balls are used. ("They could use white balls if they wanted," Berson says, "but I've never seen anyone stupid enough to do that.")

Softball is another activity that many people think is strictly for the summer. But think again. In Tawas Bay, Michigan, they play ice softball as part of the Perchville, U.S.A., festival.

Ice softball looks similar to grass surface softball until it's time to run. (Skating is not allowed as part of ice softball.)

"You can't run," says Marc Elliot, event organizer, player, and ice scraper. "It's funny watching someone new to the sport trying to take a step from the batter's box and falling flat on their fanny. It's even funnier when they keep trying to get up and they keep falling again and again."

Of course, the coldness of the season demands certain changes in the rules. For instance, games are only five innings long. Moreover, a bigger ball is used, one that can be caught with normal winter gloves, even though some insist on using baseball gloves.

If swimming in the winter cold happens to be your thing, Tawas Bay is the place to find others with the same passion. Each year, a polar bear swim is included in the local winter carnival.

"Don't know anyone today from around here who's crazy enough to jump in that cold water," says Dan Stanfield of Perchville, U.S.A. The locals, he says, content themselves with ice fishing, an endeavor that is pursued from within tiny huts constructed on the ice.

"There are dozens out there, even on the coldest of days," he says.

If heading into the winter's surf is a bit too outrageous for your tastes, there is always volleyball. But instead of sand beneath your feet, it's snow and ice beneath your boots at the Lakeside Winter Celebration in Fond du Lac, Wisconsin.

"With Wisconsin, the best season is winter," remarks event co-organizer John Geise. Some twenty-five thousand visitors come to this community to celebrate the season. "The festival helps break up the winter," he adds. "People have cabin fever, they're looking for something to do."

Events include typical winter sports such as snowmobile riding, dogsled racing, snow sculpting, and ice fishing. Then there are more unusual events—snow broomball, for instance, which is a mix of hockey and soccer played on ice with brooms and soccer balls. "Teams from all over the state come to compete," says Geise.

There's also ice bowling, which is very much like traditional bowling except for one special rule—no gutter balls. Moreover, you can bank the ball off the snow wall into the pins for a strike or spare.

The oldest and most tradition-bound of the winter events is the annual St. Paul Winter Carnival in Minnesota. It was started in 1886 to rebut an eastern journalist who had compared wintertime St. Paul to Siberia—unfit for human habitation. The Minnesotans set out to transform their cold environs into a winter wonderland, with a carnival highlighted by the construction of an ice palace 180 feet long and 106 feet high.

According to local legend, each winter during the festival a battle is waged between King Boreas, king of the cold, and Vulcanus Rex, god of heat. Actors play the roles of Boreas and Vulcan in annual parades. The grand celebration also features arts, winter sports, and antique cutter parades.

The highlight, however, remains the building of mammoth ice castles, a tradition that has recently been restored after a hiatus. Ice blocks are harvested in traditional fashion and are put in place according to intricate architectural blueprints. Many castles tower several stories into the cold winter sky.

So next time you're thinking of a January or February vacation with golf, swimming, and fishing, remember that those activities are found not only in Arizona, Florida, and California, but in the crisp, cold winter air of Michigan, Wisconsin, and Minnesota, where they truly make the most out of winter.

Event: Polar Ice Cap Golf Tournament
When: Last weekend in January
Where: Grand Haven, Michigan

Contact: Association of Commerce and Industry
1 Washington Street
Grand Haven, MI 49417
(616) 842-4910

Something about the event: Hundreds of golfers assemble to shoot 9 or 18 holes on Spring Lake, on a course carved out of the ice and snow.

Accommodations with a personal touch:
See "Tulip Time," page 101.

Roadside food: See "Tulip Time," page 101.

Some readings to enhance travels: Teale, Edwin, *Wandering through Winter*, Dodd, Mead, 1981; Alexander, Arch, *The Joy of Golf*, Pendulum Books, 1982; Armour, Tommy, *How To Play Your Best Golf Game All the Time*, Simon & Schuster, 1971; McIntosh, Jon, *Hooked On Golf*, Ipswich Press, 1982; Oman, Mark, *How To Live with a Golfaholic: A Survival Guide For Family and Friends of Passionate Players*, Golfaholics Anonymous, 1987. See also "Tulip Time," page 101.

Turn off here along the way: Grand Haven during the spring and summer is a busy port town and a mecca for visitors who favor its woods and waters. One draw to the area is the famous "singing sand" on local beaches, so named because the sand emits a whistling sound when it is walked on. During the tourist season, the town features a boardwalk, trolley rides, and a musical fountain.

To the east is Grand Rapids, hometown of the 38th president, the second largest city in Michigan and a community with a long industrial tradition. Faced with economic change, Grand Rapids has reacted with redevelopment. Highlights in town now include the **Gerald R. Ford Museum,** U.S. 131 at Pearl Street, NW, Grand Rapids, (616) 456-2674, which chronicles Mr. Ford's career and presidency.

Event: Lakeside Winter Celebration
When: Last weekend in January
Where: Fond du Lac, Wisconsin

Contact: Fond du Lac Festivals
207 North Main Street
Fond du Lac, WI 54935
(414) 923-3010

Something about the event: Fond du Lac hosts these two days of celebration to shake off the winter doldrums. There are dogsled races, weight pulls, a chili cook-off, ice bowling, broomball games, snowmobile races, three-wheeler races, and a Saturday night shindig.

Accommodations with a personal touch:
 Clarion Hotel (H), 1 North Main, Fond du Lac, WI 54935, (414) 923-3000: 135 rms, pb, $45-65; cc-AE, DC, DISC, MC, V; c-yes, s-yes, d-yes, p-ltd, Full Bkfst. Grand hotel of the 1920s, completely restored. Two restaurants, athletic club, and sauna.

 The **Farmer's Daughter Inn** (I), Route 1, Box 37, Ripon, WI 54971, (414) 748-2146: 4 rms, pb, $65; cc-no; c-yes, s-ltd, d-no, p-no, Bkfst-no. Turn-of-the-century gingerbread farm in the heart of dairy country.

Roadside food: Given Fond du Lac's lakeside location, it is not surprising that fish is popular here. Friday night is "Fish Fry Night." One local institution is **Wendt's Restaurant, on the Lake,** (414)

688-5231. A few years ago, **Countrywoods,** at the Holiday Inn, 625 Rolling Meadows Drive, (414) 923-1440, ran a special "Fondue at Fond du Lac" promotion that was a big success. Fondue, here a chocolate fondue with a number of available toppings, is now a permanent fixture in town.

Some readings to enhance travels: Andreas, Fred, and Agranoff, Ann, *Ice Palaces,* Abbeville Press, 1983; Durocher, Joseph F., *Practical Ice Carving,* Van Nostrand Reinhold, 1981; Haseqawa, Hideo, *Ice Carving,* Books for Bakers, 1978. See also "The Great Circus Parade," page 113.

Turn off here along the way: Fond du Lac, "farther end of the lake," is the name given by the French traders who originally surveyed the area. The town is symbolized by the lighthouse perched at the edge of Lake Winnebago.

The **Cathedral of St. Paul,** 51 West Davis Street, (414) 921-3363, dates back to the 1860s and features rare ecclesiastical artifacts, including a 13th-century crucifix, mosaics, and stained glass. Even older is **St. Patrick's Church,** 41 East Follett Street, (414) 921-0347, built by Irish immigrants in 1856.

The **Historic Galloy House and Village,** 336 Old Pioneer Road, (414) 922-6390, has been restored to its Victorian splendor. Around it have been placed 20 other Victorian structures that once stood in town. They include a railway depot, a schoolroom, a church, a post office, and a courtroom.

Event: Christmas Bird Count
When: Mid-December
Where: Indiana Dunes, Indiana

Contact: Christmas Bird Count
c/o 1265 Redbud Drive
Chesterton, IN 46304
(219) 926-1978

Something about the event: Indiana Dunes National Lakeshore is a little-known gem of a park situated along the shores of Lake Michigan, not far from downtown Chicago. Each year, bird lovers track the numbers of various species in and around the dunes and the park as part of a nationwide census. The event is coordinated by the Audubon Society.

Accommodations with a personal touch:
   Duneland Beach Inn (I), 3311 Potawatomi, Michigan City, IN 46360, (219) 874-7729: 10 rms, 2 pb, $35-80; cc-MC, V; c-yes, s-yes, d-no, p-no, Full Bkfst; h-Donna Fiorito. Inn near dunes has sitting room and private beach. Full breakfast. Accessible to Chicago and South Bend.
   Creekwood Inn (I), Route 20-35 at I-94, Michigan City, IN 46360, (219) 872-8357: 12 rms, pb, $85-95; cc-AE, MC, V; c-yes, s-yes, d-yes, p-no, Cont Bkfst; h-Peggy Wall. Country inn near lakefront, in wooded area, serves afternoon tea with sweets.
   The **Plantation Inn** (I), R.R. 2, Box 296S, Michigan City, IN 46360, (219) 874-2418: 5 rms, pb, $60-75; cc-AE, MC, V; c-ltd, s-yes, d-no, p-ltd, Full Bkfst; h-Ann Stephens. Southern-style plantation two miles from lake.

Roadside food: Lobsters are flown in daily to **Maxine Heine,** 521 Franklin Square, Michigan City, (219) 879-9068. Prime ribs are also on the nightly menu. The place is described as having "a little something for everyone." The **Hunter Restaurant,** 3311 Potawatomi Trail, Michigan City, (219) 874-7729, features French and American cuisine, including local fish and fowl, and fresh local fruit such as raspberries and peaches when in season. It's a drive but a scenic one to good seafood and lake fish at **Miller's Country House,** along the shore of Lake Michigan at 16409 Red Arrow Highway, Union Pier, MI 49129, (616) 469-5950.

Some readings to enhance travels: Daniel, Glenda, *Dune Country: A Guide for Hikers and Naturalists,* Swallow, 1977; Keller, Charles E., et al., *Indiana Birds and Their Haunts: A Checklist and Finding Guide,* 2d ed., Indiana University Press, 1986; Mumford, Russell, and Keller, Charles E., *The Birds of Indiana,* Indiana University Press, 1984; Starling, Alfred, *Enjoying Indiana Birds,* Indiana University Press, 1978. See also "500 Festival," page 102.

Turn off here along the way: Michigan City is considered a leading lakeside resort because of its proximity to both the dunes and Chicago. Winter is not the prime tourist season; nonetheless, the shoreline holds its own special beauty at that time.
   One place worth a visit at any time of year is the **Barker Civic Center,** 631 Washington Street, (219) 873-1520, a 38-room mansion containing furnishings and artifacts from the turn of the century.
   The beauty of the Indiana Dunes becomes even more remarkable if one travels just a bit to the west, to the giant industrial city of Gary, one of the centers of American steel. There, and at

nearby Hammond, one is struck by the scale of the operations. One is also struck by the vast lands of former industry that now lie abandoned, a witness to the industry's heyday that stretches back to 1905 in Gary.

To the east, the legends of the Gipper and Knute Rockne live on at the **University of Notre Dame,** which is renowned for its educational programs and its football traditions.

Event: International Pancake Race
When: Shrove Tuesday (day before Ash Wednesday)
Where: Liberal, Kansas

Contact: International Pancake Race
Pancake Board
P.O. Box 665
Liberal, KS 67901
(316) 624-1106

Something about the event: The pancake race is a Shrove Tuesday tradition in England. The Kansas contest, established in 1950, brings together women from Liberal and their counterparts from the English town of Olney, where the tradition dates back to 1445. They run a quarter-mile course with skillets in their hands, flipping pancakes as they go.

Accommodations with a personal touch:
Hardesty House (I), 712 Main Street, Ashland, KS 67831, (316) 635-2911: 10 rms, pb, $24.95-$29.95; cc-AE, MC, V; c-yes, s-yes, d-no, p-no, Cont Bkfst (also evening meal). Turn-of-the-century hotel a drive to the east from Liberal. Period furnishings, including an oil stove, hanging kerosene lamps, and pictures that chronicle Ashland's history.

The **Cimarron Hotel and Restaurant** (H), 203 North Main Street, Cimarron, KS 67835, (318) 855-2244: 9 rms, pb-no, $20-30; cc-no; c-yes, s-yes, d-no, p-yes, Full Bkfst; h-Kathleen Holt. Restored trail and railroad hotel dating back to 1887 is now a registered National Historic Landmark decorated in period style. All rooms overlook Main Street.

Roadside food: If those runners with pancakes have made you hungry, you might head to the **Pancake House,** 640 East Pancake Street, (316) 624-8585, to eat some—yup—pancakes.

Some readings to enhance travels: Davis, Kenneth S., *Kansas*, Norton, 1976; Federal Writers' Project, American Guide Series, *Kansas: A Guide to the Sunflower State*, Hastings, 1958; Zornow, William F., *Kansas: A History of the Jayhawk State*, University of Oklahoma Press, 1971.

Ashby, Susan P., *Pancakes from Vinegar Hill Farm*, Winston-Derel, 1984; Brent, Carol D., *Pancakes-Waffles: The Fine Art of Pancake, Waffle, Crepe and Blintz*, T-T Recipe, 1970; Anderson, Bob, ed., *Complete Runner*, Anderson World, 1982.

Turn off here along the way: You can learn about what life was like in Liberal (before pancakes) at the **Coronado Museum,** 567 East Cedar Street, (316) 624-7624, which explores the history of Kansas back to pioneer times. Next door is a replica of **Dorothy's House,** from *The Wizard of Oz,* (316) 624-7624. You can see film clips from the legendary movie there.

Another Liberal sight is **"Mighty Sampson,"** a 1200-foot-long natural bridge that towers 100 feet above the Cimarron River.

Liberal lies just north of the Kansas–Oklahoma border. Fifty miles to the northwest is Dodge City, of frontier fame.

CENTRAL

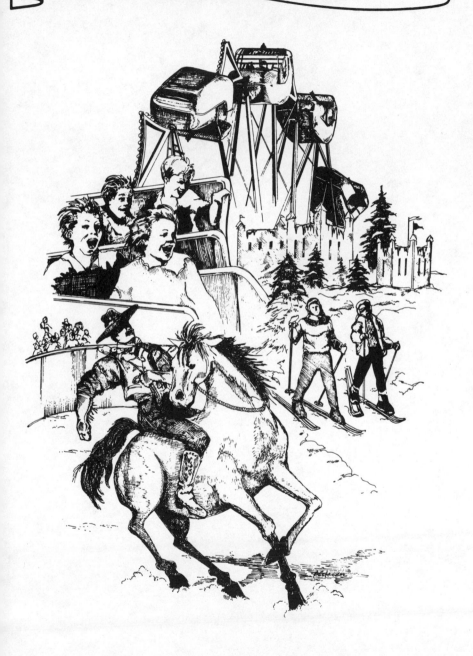

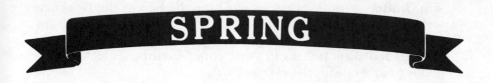

SPRING

Turning Back the Clock on American Transportation

It's early morning at the Victorian-era train terminal. A crowd works its way past the stained-glass ceiling and the arched roofs toward Track 8. At trackside lie Pullman coaches built in 1917. The train is packed. A whistle blows.

It's not rush hour, and this isn't a group of commuters. The folks packing the train are about to embark on an eight-hour, 170-mile old-time train trip.

Old-time transportation is big business these days. Events and trips are held year-round and nationwide. After years of unimpeded "progress" on the tracks and roads and in the skies, many people have come to realize that getting there is indeed half the fun.

On this particular Sunday, the train belongs to the Blue Mountain and Reading Railroad, one of several companies that have set out to revive the railroad tradition. The Pullman cars are pulled by a mid-1940s steam engine, the 2102, one of only three still in existence. Its physical statistics are as impressive as its classic looks: It is 110 feet long and weighs 441,300 pounds, including 19,000 pounds of water and 26 tons of coal needed to run the engine.

And of course, there is the sound of the whistle, magically echoing in the air.

On board, there's a mixed group, led by the hard-core rail fans, well furnished with buttons, hats, T-shirts, maps, books, even walkie-talkies. The rest of the group are plain folks out for a ride; men and women, young and old, trying to get a sense of the engines and passenger cars of yesteryear.

The train trip recalls not just an earlier era in transporation, but a different way of life. The railroad helped build communities and served as the focal point of many a town. One such community was Grafton, West Virginia, at one time the hub of the Baltimore and Ohio rail system, which spanned the Appalachians and transported both passengers and goods. Grafton was a railroad town. Sons joined their fathers in what could then be expected to be lifelong careers with the railroad.

Eventually, the B&O was replaced by Amtrak, service deteriorated, the passenger train route was shut down, and the old station was closed.

Once a year Grafton recalls its proud history at the Railroad Heritage Festival. Restored passenger cars from the 1936–1941 era are brought back to life again for a weekend. The crowd enjoys railroad memorabilia, music, foods, crafts, and street entertainment.

"We're trying to keep an area railroad heritage alive," says Sherman Davidson, a festival organizer. "Kids growing up here today never see a regularly scheduled passenger train. Because of our history it is important for them to see how important the railroad was to the town."

At the Golden Spike National Historic Site in Promontory, Utah, there is an annual reenactment of the completion on May 10, 1869, of the transcontinental railroad. (See "Golden Spike Reenactment," page 140.) The day is commemorated by the "wedding of the engines" at the site and by speeches honoring the twenty thousand workers—mostly Irish, Italian, German, and Chinese immigrants— who built the 1,776-mile railroad over a 30-year period. The crowd assembles in period costumes to watch the Union Pacific engine from the east and the Central Pacific engine from the west meet again to symbolically make the nation one.

In August, the National Historic Park, in Promontory, hosts an annual Railroader's Festival that demonstrates how the coming of the railroad changed the West.

It was first the automobile and then the airplane that drew passengers away from the rails in the mid-20th century. But in recent years the rails have made a comeback of sorts in the form of the trolley.

Only a few decades ago, more than one hundred thousand trolley cars crisscrossed American cities. Track and wire were part of the urban landscape. (In fact, the Brooklyn baseball club was named the Trolley Dodgers, afterward shortened to Dodgers, because Brooklynites were renowned for artfully avoiding the numerous trolleys that careened over their streets. The Dodgers kept their name when they moved to Los Angeles, by then the home of the freeway.) But as Americans started buying cars, the perceived to be slow and noisy trolleys were abandoned.

Their decline was hastened by a company called National City Lines, which bought and dismantled many city trolley systems after World War II. It has now been documented that the firm was backed by General Motors, Standard Oil of California, rubber companies, and others with an interest in promoting the automobile. By the 1970s, the trolley was but a memory in North America. The car was king. The young, the old, and the poor had to make do with buses.

Paradoxically, the success of the automobile—and the problems associated with it (i.e., pollution and congestion)—has caused a resurgence of interest in trolleys. These days, they are euphemistically called Light Rapid Transit (LRT). Portland and Los Angeles are installing new systems on the rights-of-way where trolleys once ran. San Diego and Sacramento have successfully launched new systems. A few fortunate communities that never quite found the money, political will, or callousness to destroy their trolley systems—including New Orleans, Pittsburgh, Boston, and Philadelphia—have restored and upgraded them.

San Francisco has the most famous street railroad. Those little cable cars that Tony Bennett described as going halfway to the stars have been repaired and are fully back in service. (Actually, cable cars and trolleys are not the same. Cable cars are engineless, pulled by mechanized cables; trolleys have electric motors that run on power supplied by overhead wires.) The city hosts the annual Cable Car Bell Ringing Competition. Ray Rezzos, a gripman on the Municipal Railway, says of bell ringing, "It's a real art, because all bells are different."

"Some ropes hold tight, allowing one ring at a time," he explained. "The best rope will hold loose enough to allow the bell to jiggle, and a good ringer can get the bell to ring four or five times for just one pull."

Cable cars are but one aspect of the history of the trolley in the Bay City. Each summer San Francisco honors its past and the past of trolley travel throughout the world with the annual Trolley Festival. Vehicles come from as far away as Hamburg, West Germany (the Red Baron), and Melbourne, Australia.

A redevelopment project on Market Street downtown has "derailed" the Trolley Festival, at least temporarily. But upon completion of the project, the trolley will run down Market, along the waterfront, reaching a terminus at Fisherman's Wharf. The Trolley Festival is expected to resume after the extension is completed.

Although it has taken almost four decades, it appears we've finally gotten back on the tracks.

Event: Anniversary of Golden
Spike Ceremony Reenactment
When: May 10
Where: Promontory, Utah

Contact: Golden Spike National Historic Site
P.O. Box W
Brigham City, UT 84302
(801) 471-2209

Something about the event: The construction of the transcontinental railroad was completed in 1869. To mark the occasion, a golden railroad spike was driven into the ties at the point where the Union Pacific and Central Pacific lines met. The event is reenacted with period costumes and engines.

Accommodations with a personal touch:
   Center Street Bed and Breakfast (B&B), 169 East Center Street, Logan, UT 84321, (801) 752-3443: 9 rms, 5 pb, $20-70; cc-MC, V; c-ltd, s-no, d-yes, p-no, Cont Bkfst. Home and carriage house located in the Cache Valley.
   Bed 'n Breakfast Association of Utah (S), P.O. Box 16465, Salt Lake City, UT 84116, (801) 532-7076.

Roadside food: Steaks, chicken steaks, home-cooked food, and homemade pies are the highlights at the **Ox Ranch House,** 1900 Highway 89, Perry, (801) 544-5474. A longtime family restaurant is the **Idle Isle,** 24 South Main Street, Brigham City, (801) 734-9062. The food, desserts, and even the candy are all homemade. Casual western-style dining may be found at the **Western Trails Cafe,** 59 West Main Street, Tremont, (801) 257-3323. Highlights are "Utah-style" chili, with beans and meat, and pastries made in the kitchen.

Some readings to enhance travels: Peters, Charles S., *Utah,* Norton, 1977; Poll, Richard D., *Utah's History,* Brigham Young University Press, 1978; Roylance, Ward J., *Utah: A Guide to the State,* Western Epics, 1982.
   DeGolyer, Everett L., Jr., *The Track Going Back: A Century of the Transcontinental Railroad, 1869–1969,* Amon Carter Museum of Western Art, 1979; Drury, George, *Historical Guide to North American Railroads,* Kalmbach, 1986; Dafua, Thamar E., *Transcontinental Railroad Legislation, 1835–1862,* Ayer, 1981; Fulton, Robert L., *Epic of the Overland: An Account of the Building of the Central and*

Union Pacific Railroad, Borogo Press, 1982; Reeder, Clarence A., Jr., *The History of Utah's Railroads, 1869–1883,* Ayer, 1981; Robertson, Donald B., *Encyclopedia of Western Railroad History: The Western States,* Caxton, 1986.

Turn off here along the way: The Visitor Center at the **Golden Spike National Historic Site,** (801) 471-2209, describes the building and operation of the transcontinental railroad.

Brigham City, to the east, is named after the early Mormon leader Brigham Young. The influence of both the railroad and the Mormon Church are seen at the **Brigham City Museum and Gallery,** 24 North 300 West, (801) 723-6769.

On a clear day, **Inspiration Point** offers a panoramic view of the area and beyond for miles.

To the south, along I-15, is Ogden. It too has a history dominated by the rails and the Mormon Church. It became a major switching point on the railroad soon after the transcontinental connection was made. Non-worshipers are not permitted inside the **Ogden Tabernacle and Temple,** but can gaze from outside along 2133 Washington Boulevard.

Event: Horseback Endurance Ride
When: Second weekend in April
Where: Hurricane, Utah

Contact: Endurance Ride
P.O. Box 101
Hurricane, UT 84737
(801) 635-4627

Something about the event: Horseback teams from Utah, Nebraska, California, and Colorado compete in 25- and 50-mile races.

Accommodations with a personal touch:

Green Gate Village Bed and Breakfast (B&B), 62-78 West Tabernacle, St. George, UT 84770, (801) 628-6999: 15 rms, pb, $35-100 couple ($10 each additional); cc-MC, V; c-yes, s-no, d-ltd, p-ltd, Full Bkfst; h-Shanna Rae Durfey. Historic building with period furniture and authentic antiques. Historic buildings nearby.

Seven Wives Inn (I), 217 North 100 West, St. George, UT 84770, (801) 628-3737: 12 rms, pb, $25-65; cc-DISC, MC, V; c-yes, s-no, d-ltd, p-yes, Full Bkfst; h-Jay and Donna Curtis. The seven wives were married to the owner's great-grandfather back when Mormons still practiced polygamy. Inn, built circa 1833, is on the National Historic Register.

Zion House Bed and Breakfast (B&B), 801 Zion Park Boulevard, Springdale, UT 84767, (801) 772-3281: 3 rms, pb-1, $33-39 ($8 each additional person); cc-no; c-over 12, s-no, d-no, p-no, Full Bkfst; h-Lellie and Alan Baiardi. Inn, surrounded by peaks of Zion National Park, features comfortable living room and library.

Under the Eaves Guest House (B&B), P.O. Box 29, Springdale, UT 84767, (801) 772-3457: 3 rms, 1 pb, $35-65; cc-MC, V; c-yes, s-no, d-yes, p-yes, Full Bkfst; h-Kathleen Brown. English cottage guest house, surrounded by national park, was built, but never used, as a post office. Early western furnishings and antiques.

Roadside food: The **Bitten Spur Restaurant,** 1212 Zion Boulevard, Springdale, (801) 772-3498, has such a reputation for good Sonoran Mexican food that folks are known to drive for three hours just to come there for dinner. **Andolin's,** 290 East St. George Boulevard, St. George, (801) 673-5152, specializes in Old English cuisine such as prime ribs and brisket. **Dick's Cafe,** 114 Boulevard East in St. George, (801) 673-3841, is the place to tank up with coffee and find out the local news.

Some readings to enhance travels: Faragher, John M., *Women and Men on the Overland Trail,* Yale University Press, 1979; Heap, Gwenn H., *Central Route to the Pacific,* Ayer, 1981. (See also "Anniversary of Golden Spike Ceremony," page 140.)

Turn off here along the way: The **Hurricane Fault,** a jagged escarpment rising 7,000 feet over town, is the source of the town's name. Hurricane is home to the world's largest natural hot springs, **Pah Tempe Springs,** S.R. 9, Hurricane, (801) 635-2879.

St. George, to the west on Route 29, has a number of pioneer and Mormon displays, including **Daughters of Pioneers Museum,** 143 North 100 East Street.

The biggest draw of southern Utah is its scenery. **Zion National Park,** (801) 772-3256, and **Bryce Canyon State Park,** (801) 834-5322, are paradises for hikers and photographers. Bryce Canyon features sandstone canyon walls and geological formations from lava flows centuries ago.

Event: Festival of Nations
When: Last weekend in April
Where: St. Paul, Minnesota

Contact: International Institute of Minnesota
1694 Como Avenue
St. Paul, Minnesota 55108
(612) 647-0191

Something about the event: Three day event, sponsored by the International Institute of Minnesota, features 6,000 people representing 55 ethnic groups. Activities include dance, music, crafts, an international bazaar, and countless varieties of food. A special highlight is a stage offering continuous entertainment.

Accommodations with a personal touch:

Chatsworth Bed and Breakfast (B&B), 984 Ashland, St. Paul, MN 55104, (612) 227-4288: 5 rms, 2 pb, $42-85; cc-no; c-ltd, s-no, d-no, p-no, Cont-Plus Bkfst; h-Donna Gustafson. Turn-of-the-century Victorian home decorated in international theme. Situated in heart of St. Paul, near governor's mansion.

Thorwood (I), Fourth and Pine, Hastings, MN 55033, (612) 437-3297: 7 rms, pb, $65-125; cc-AE, MC, V; c-ltd, s-ltd, d-no, p-no, Full Bkfst. French Second Empire home from 1880s, half an hour's drive to St. Paul. Large rooms with dining areas in each. Local wine with evening snacks. Situated one block from the Mississippi River bluff.

River Town Inn (I), 306 West Olive Street, Stillwater, MN 55082, (612) 430-2955: 9 rms, pb, $45-115; cc-MC, V; c-no, s-no, d-no, p-no, Full Bkfst; h-Judy and Chuck Dougherty. One of Minnesota's oldest inns. Rooms with fireplaces, Victorian antiques, and whirlpools.

St. Paul Hotel (H), 350 Market Street, St. Paul, MN 55102, (612) 292-9292: 254 rms, pb, $94-240; cc-AE, MC, V; c-yes, s-yes, d-yes, p-no, Bkfst-no. Historic hotel from 1910, situated in downtown St. Paul.

Nicollet Island Inn (I), 95 Merriam, Nicollet Island, Minneapolis, MN 55401, (612) 623-7741: 24 rms, pb, $50-75; cc-AE, DC, MC, V; c-yes, s-yes, d-no, p-no, Cont Bkfst (also lunch and dinner); h-Philip Arensen. Restored inn, circa 1893, situated along the Mississippi River.

Roadside food: The Festival of Nations is a meeting of cultures, and on Grand Avenue in St. Paul you can find Italian, Chinese, Afghan, and South American restaurants. Still, the fact is that the Twin Cities have mainly been molded by the Scandinavian emigrant presence. At the **Willows,** in the Hyatt Regency Hotel, 1300 Nicollet Mall, Minneapolis, (612) 370-1234, the chef prepares a Scandinavian specialty every day. Also on the menu are seafood, veal, chicken, and lamb. The **Loon Cafe,** 500 First Avenue North, Minneapolis, (612) 332-8342, is a good spot to warm up in a friendly Minneapolis atmosphere. The menu features soup, salad, sandwiches, and five kinds of chili. If you're willing to drive some distance away, you can taste the legendary Norwegian lutefisk at **Crabtree's Kitchen,** Route 95, Marine on St. Croix, MN, (612) 433-2455. Other features are lefse bread and Swedish sausage.

Some readings to enhance travels: Blegen, Theodore C., *Minnesota, A History of the State,* University of Minnesota Press, 1963; Lass, William E., *Minnesota,* Norton, 1977; Olsenius, Richard, *Minnesota Travel Companion,* Blumstem, 1983.

Ervin, Jean, *The Twin Cities Perceived,* University of Minnesota Press, 1976; Koeper, H. E., *Historic St. Paul Buildings,* St. Paul City Planning Board, 1964; Sandeen, Ernst, *St. Paul's Historic Summit Avenue,* Macalaster College, 1978.

De Vos, George, and Romanucci-Ross, Lola, *Ethnic Identity: Cultural Continuities and Change,* Mayford, 1975; Morrison, Joan, and Zabusky, Charlotte Fox, *American Mosaic,* Dutton, 1955; Williams, William Carlos, *In the American Grain,* New Directions, 1956.

Turn off here along the way: Once you're done at the festival, there's still lots to keep you occupied in St. Paul. Minnesota's state capital is the less publicized half of the Twin Cities. It is part of a big city, yet it maintains a small-town ambience.

The first landmark one is likely to notice is the **Cathedral of St. Paul,** 239 Shelby Avenue, (612) 225-6563. Styled after St. Peter's Basilica in Rome, it has been a magnet for immigrants for generations.

Not far away is the **State Capitol,** University Avenue between Wabasha and Cedar, (612) 297-3521, whose cornerstone was laid in 1898. More than 25 varieties of granite were used in its construction. It has one of the largest unsupported domes in the country.

You can find drama and music at the **Crawford Theatre, Landmark Center,** 75 West Fifth Street, (612) 292-3225, and the **Ordway Theatre,** 345 Washington Street, (612) 224-4222.

The **Science Museum of Minnesota,** 30 East Tenth Street, (612) 221-9400, presents programs on space and science. It has a domed overhead screen, one of only a few worldwide.

The **World Theatre,** 10 East Exchange, (612) 298-1222, once hosted "A Prairie Home Companion."

Of course, there is a whole other world on the Minneapolis side of the Mississippi. (See "St. Paul Winter Carnival," page 175.)

Event: 89er Days
When: Mid-April
Where: Guthrie, Oklahoma

Contact: Chamber of Commerce
Box 995
Guthrie, OK 73044
(405) 282-1947

Something about the event: The Oklahoma Territory was opened for settlement on April 22, 1889. To commemorate the famous rush for land, Guthrie hosts rodeos, carnivals, parades, crafts, and a chuck-wagon feed.

Accommodations with a personal touch:

Flora's Bed and Breakfast (B&B), 2312 Northwest 46th, Oklahoma City, OK 73112, (405) 840-3157: 2 rms, pb, $30-35; cc-no; c-ltd, s-yes, d-yes, p-no, Cont Bkfst; h-Joanne Flora. B&B, accessible to downtown, built into side of hill. Antique-filled rooms.

The **Grandison** (I), 1841 Northwest 15th, Oklahoma City, OK 73106, (405) 521-0011: 6 rms, pb, $35-90; cc-no; c-over 12, s-ltd, d-yes, p-no, Cont Bkfst; h-Bob and Claudia Wright. Inn was built before Oklahoma was a state. A 1919 addition includes stained glass and original brass fixtures.

Roadside food: As in much of the south and west, barbecue is king here. A popular barbecue eatery in town is **Stables Cafe,** 223 North Division, (405) 282-0893. Home-style chicken-fried steaks are served at **Territorial House,** 224 North Division, (405) 282-6733.

Some readings to enhance travels: Gibson, Arrell M., *The History of Oklahoma,* University of Oklahoma Press, 1984; McReynolds, Edwin, *Oklahoma,* University of Oklahoma Press, 1969; Morgan, H. Wayne and Anne H. G., *Oklahoma: A History,* Norton, 1984; Ruth, Kent, *Oklahoma Travel Handbook,* University of Oklahoma Press, 1977; Wilson, Steve, *Oklahoma Treasures and Treasure Tales,* University of Oklahoma Press, 1976; Federal Writers' Project, American Guide Series, *Oklahoma: A Guide to the Sooner State*, Somerset, 1938; Erickson, John R., *Panhandle Cowboy*, University of Nebraska Press, 1980.

Turn off here along the way: Guthrie was Oklahoma's first capital, from 1907 to 1910. Oklahoma's beginnings are recalled at the **Territorial Museum**, 402 East Oklahoma Avenue, (405) 282-1889, a turn-of-the-century building with ornate and intricate architectural details, down to the grilles and radiators. An exhibit describes the printing of Oklahoma's first newspaper.

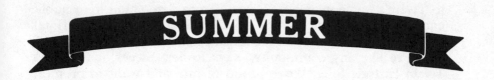

SUMMER

Celebrating Literary America

In an age of television, the very notion of a festival devoted to a writer may be considered cause for celebration. After all, we are often reminded how little anyone reads any more.

Literary festivals, while not commonplace, do appear on events calendars nationwide. Many a town has embraced a "favorite son" (or daughter) years after the writer's death. Sometimes there is an ironic twist to this relationship, as when the writer had a troubled or problematic experience there.

The name of Samuel Clemens, popularly known as Mark Twain, is inextricably linked to the small Missouri town of Hannibal, which lies along the banks of the Mississippi River (See "Tom Sawyer Days," page 110). His childhood in the town and along the river served as inspiration for his most famous works, *The Adventures of Tom Sawyer* and *The Adventures of Huckleberry Finn,* as well as his memoir *Life on the Mississippi.* Reporter, raconteur, and critic of the American scene, Twain captured the essence of the American experience in the 19th century. To many around the world, Mark Twain is the epitome of American literature.

However, none of Twain's books were written in Missouri. He left Hannibal for good at the age of 17, spent some years as a steamboat pilot on the Mississippi, then became a roving journalist for a series of newspapers, traveling through the country and abroad. Twain did most of his mature writing while living in Hartford, Connecticut.

Twain's upbringing and his wanderings made him a tough-edged but eloquent individual who cultivated an earthy persona. Some of his best satire and social criticism made use of his memories of Hannibal. As his fame grew, so did the town's reputation. Today, the Twain connection is felt throughout Hannibal. In addition to Twain's home, which was saved from demolition by a public campaign in 1912, one may also find the Mark Twain Motor Hotel, Mark Twain Antiques, and the Huck Finn Shopping Center.

"We're like any community," says Robert Sweet of the Mark Twain Historic Site. "We're proud of him and want to promote our specialness."

In contrast to Twain, Sinclair Lewis was notorious in his home town, and was rarely seen as a hero during his lifetime. In his novels, Lewis portrayed the narrowness of small-town life. Although the town in his famous *Main Street* was named Gopher Prairie, it is clear that he had his hometown of Sauk Centre, Minnesota, in mind.

The residents of Sauk Centre considered the portrayal an insult. A sign installed some years ago outside Lewis's house rationalized the matter, calling him "a gawky sensitive child, who achieved success in school and was the brunt of every cruel piece of horseplay . . ."

These days, most townfolk are not bitter. "Few in town now actually remember him personally," says Betty Smith of the Chamber of Commerce. But there are still those who make a fuss. Many are involved in a group called the Sinclair Lewis Interpretive Center, a name that says a lot about the impact of the writer's criticisms on his neighbors. In addition to providing community group therapy of sorts (by helping the town to come to grips with Lewis's writings), the center assists visitors. Folks at the center will direct you to the Lewis Museum, his boyhood home, his grave site, and to a restored hotel where he worked. And, of course, they'll also point out Main Street.

It is hard to find anyone in Sauk Centre who still expresses outrage toward Lewis. The town today seems to harbor a large number of Lewis junkies who can recite information on any aspect of his life and work. Some, of course, might have despised Lewis had they lived at the time his books were published. But because Lewis now generates tourist dollars, they endorse, or at least tolerate, Lewis for the good of the town.

Sinclair Lewis's birthday has even replaced July Fourth as a time to celebrate in Sauk Centre. Independence Day in town is a quiet time. Instead, they save the parade and fireworks for the next week, when they hold the annual Sinclair Lewis Days (see page 149).

The relationship between John Steinbeck and his neighbors in Salinas, California, was not always a warm one. His neighbors did not take kindly to his portrayal of them in *The Grapes of Wrath* and other works. But today Salinas boasts the Steinbeck Library and hosts the John Steinbeck Days in July and August.

Edgar Allen Poe, while neglected and abandoned in life, is remembered every January at his grave site in Baltimore. Robert Frost has been claimed by Ripton, Vermont, even though he did not spend much of his life there. A similar connection has sprung up between Key West, Florida, and Ernest Hemingway (see "Hemingway Days," page 73).

Along with the celebrations and parades, one hopes that such communities continue to maintain archival records, so that the true relationship between writer and hometown, not just the legend, may be always recalled.

Event: Sinclair Lewis Days
When: End of June or second week in July
Where: Sauk Centre, Minnesota

Contact: Chamber of Commerce
P.O. Box 222
Sauk Centre, MN 56378
(612) 352-5201

Something about the event: Events include an auto show, swap meet, high school band concert, flea market, art show, chess tournament, soap box derby, parade, and Lewis readings.

Accommodations with a personal touch:
  Palmer House Hotel (H), 500 Sinclair Lewis Avenue, Sauk Centre, MN 56378, (612) 352-3431: 37 rms, 4 pb, $16-38; cc-no; c-yes, s-yes, d-no, p-no, Bkfst-no; h-Dick Schwartz and Al Tingley. Sinclair Lewis once worked here; he was fired for daydreaming. Many rooms have been restored and have original furnishings.

Roadside food: Dining has a distinctively old-time ambience at the restored **Palmer House Hotel** (see Accommodations). The **River's Edge Restaurant,** 26 12th Street South, (612) 352-6505, is recommended for the steak on its varied menu.

Some readings to enhance travels: Dolley, D. J., *The Art of Sinclair Lewis,* University of Nebraska Press, 1967; Fleming, Robert and Esther, *Sinclair Lewis: A Reference Guide,* G. K. Hall, 1980; Koblas, John J., *Sinclair Lewis, Home at Last,* Voyageur Press, 1981. See also "Festival of Nations," page 175.

Turn off here along the way: St. Joseph is the home of the largest community of Benedictine nuns in the world, **St. Benedict's Convent,** Minnesota Street (off I-94), (612) 362-5100. It has an authentic German organ.

There is also a Benedictine monastery, **St. John's Abbey and University,** (612) 363-2011, along Lake Sagatazan in the granite city of St. Cloud.

Event: Days of '47 Pioneer Celebration
When: Third and fourth week in July
Where: Salt Lake City, Utah

Contact: Salt Lake City Chamber of Commerce
175 East 400 Street
Salt Lake City, UT 84111
(801) 364-3631

Something about the event: This regional celebration, commemorating the settling of the area by the Mormon pioneers in 1847, features parades, pageants, music, and fireworks.

Accommodations with a personal touch:
    The Spruces Bed and Breakfast (B&B), 6151 South 900 East, Salt Lake City, UT 84121, (801) 268-8762: 4 rms, pb, $40-80; cc-AE, MC, V; c-yes, s-no, d-yes, p-no, Cont Bkfst; h-Lisa and Glenn Dutton. Gothic Victorian B&B surrounded by breeding farms.
    National Historic Bed and Breakfast of Salt Lake City (B&B), 936 East 1700 South, Salt Lake City, UT 84105, (801) 485-3535: 5 rms, 3 pb, $47-77; cc-AE, MC, V; c-over 12, s-no, d-no, p-no, Cont Bkfst; h-Mike and Katie Bartholomew. Remodeled Victorian home from 1890s. Features 1950s diner with jukebox that plays period tunes.
    Pinecrest Bed and Breakfast Inn (B&B), 6211 Emigration Canyon, Salt Lake City, UT 84108, (801) 583-6663: 6 rms, pb, $55-140; cc-AE, MC, V; c-yes, s-yes, d-no, p-no, Full Bkfst; h-Phil Davis. Inn, built in 1915 with stone from nearby quarry, is on six acres of landscaped gardens in the midst of wooded canyons.
    Saltair Bed and Breakfast (B&B), 164 South Ninth East, Salt Lake City, UT 84102, (801) 533-8184: 5 rms, 2 pb, $29-59; cc-MC, V; c-ltd, s-no, d-no, p-no, Cont Bkfst; h-Jan Bartlett and Nancy Saxton. Inn, built in 1903, is listed on National Historic Register. Antiques, central location.

Bed and Breakfast Homestay of Utah (S), P.O. Box 355, Salt Lake City, UT 84110, (801) 532-7076.

Roadside food: Prime ribs are served at **Diamond Lil's,** 1528 West North Temple, (801) 533-0547. **Lamb's Greek Cafe,** 169 Main Street, (801) 364-7166, features liver and onions and rice pudding in addition to traditional favorites such as steak, lamb chops, and Utah trout. The restaurant has been a family business for 70 years and has won an award for its coffee. Prime ribs, seafood, and chicken are served in a unique setting in the **Old South City Jail Restaurant,** 460 South 1000 East, (801) 355-2422.

Some readings to enhance travels: Dunbar, Seymour, *History of Travel in America,* 4 vols., Greenwood, 1968 (reprint of 1918 ed.); Holmes, Kenneth L., ed., *Covered Wagon Women: Diaries and Other Letters from the Western Trails, 1840–1849,* A. H. Clark, 1983; Nash, Roderick, *Wilderness and the American Mind,* Yale University Press, 1982. See also "Anniversary of Golden Spike Celebration," page 140.

Turn off here along the way: In Utah, the word "pioneers" means the Mormon settlers who came to the wilderness in 1847 to set up a new Zion. Secular and religious history are closely intertwined here. Salt Lake City remains the headquarters of the Mormon Church (formally known as the Church of Jesus Christ of Latter-day Saints).

Of course, the biggest draw in Salt Lake City is **Temple Square,** where both the **Temple** and the **Tabernacle** (801) 531-2534, are located. Tours are available.

Pioneer Trail State Park, (801) 533-5881, occupies the site where the Mormons first entered the valley. The park exhibits pioneer homes ranging from adobe huts and log cabins through Mormon leader Brigham Young's farmhouse.

The **Pioneer Craft House,** 3271 South 500 East Street, (801) 467-6611, is a school and museum founded during the centennial of the migration in 1947. It features crafts of Utah.

The **Utah Historical Society,** 300 Rio Grande, (801) 533-5755, is best known for the restored railroad station and the 1880s train in its collection. It also presents the history of non-Mormon groups in the area. The State Capitol, Capitol Hill, offers an overview of town. Tours of the marble and granite structure, featuring rotundas and ceiling murals, are available. For more information, call (801) 533-5900.

Event: Texas Folklife Festival
When: First weekend in August
Where: San Antonio, Texas

Contact: Institute of Texan Cultures
P.O. Box 1226
San Antonio, TX 78294
(512) 226-7651

Something about the event: Six thousand people representing 30 groups come together at the Hemisfair Plaza to celebrate the state's ethnic diversity and pioneer heritage with a celebration of their traditions, crafts, food, and dance. Activities include roping and shingle-splitting. The contemporary ethnic foods range from Hungarian gulyas to Filipino lumpia.

Accommodations with a personal touch:
Menger Hotel (H), 204 Alamo Plaza, San Antonio, TX 78205, (512) 223-4361: 325 rms, pb, $68-90; cc-AE, MC, V; c-yes, s-yes, d-yes, p-yes, Bkfst-no. Historic hotel dating back to 1859 has been restored to original interior.

The **Bullis** (I), 621 Pierce Street, P.O. Box 8059, San Antonio, TX 78208, (512) 223-9426: 9 rms, 1 pb, $24-49; cc-AE, DC, MC, V; c-yes, s-yes, d-no, p-no, Cont Bkfst; h-Alma Cross. Inn, built in 1908 for General Bullis, has Victorian decor.

Bed and Breakfast Hosts of San Antonio Home Lodging Service (S), 66 Rockhill, San Antonio, TX 78209, (512) 824-8036.

Roadside food: San Antonio provides a variety of eating opportunities, especially along the restored riverfront area. Mexican food plays a prominent role. **Margarita's,** 5811 Culebra, (512) 434-4977, features fajitas and tacos. **Casa Rio,** 430 East Commerce, (512) 225-6718, specializes in Carne Asada, charcoaled beef tenderized in tomato sauce, along with rice and refried beans. **Michelino's,** 521 River Walk, (512) 223-2939, offers Italian specialties, notably fettucine and chicken Italiana.

Some readings to enhance travels: Berry, Pat, *Lone Star: A Celebration of Texas,* Texas Monthly Press, 1977; Federal Writers' Project, American Guide Series, *Texas: A Guide to the Lone Star State,* rev. ed., Hastings, 1969; Fehrenbach, T. R., *Lone Star: A History of Texas and the Texans,* Macmillan, 1980; Fischer, John, *From the High Plains,* Harper, 1980; Frantz, Joe B., *Texas,* Norton, 1976; Kent, Rosemary, *The Genuine Texas Handbook,* Workman, 1981.

Abernathy, Francis E., ed., *T for Texas*, E-Heart Press Inc., 1982; Bauman, Richard, and Abrahams, Rose D., *And Other Neighborly Races: Social Process and Cultural Image in Texas Folklore*, University of Texas Press, 1981; Boatright, Moody, *Texas Folk and Folklore*, Southern Methodist University Press, 1954; O'Connor, Robert F., ed., *Texas Myths*, Texas A&M University Press, 1966; Patrick, M., *Texas Lore*, Red Rose Studio, 1985.

Turn off here along the way: Unlike Dallas and Houston, San Antonio is a vibrant city that hasn't lost its roots.

The best-known building in San Antonio is the **Alamo,** where a small group of Texan rebels were wiped out by Mexican forces in 1836. Though the battle was lost, the cry "Remember the Alamo!" spurred the Texan army on to win independence from Mexico. Now part of the city's downtown district, the Alamo, (512) 225-1391, houses two historical museums.

The impact of the Alamo has been felt in San Antonio's history since. For example, it is where Teddy Roosevelt's Rough Riders were formed in 1898 following Spain's attack on the U.S.S. *Maine* in Havana harbor.

The **Buckhorn Hall of Horns Museum** on U.S. 281, (512) 226-8301, is a gallery of animal horns and antlers and stuffed wildlife.

The site of the festival, Hemisfair Plaza, 600 Hemisfair Park, is also home to the **Texas Science Center,** (512) 226-5544, and the **Tower of the Americas,** a concrete structure 662 feet tall. There is a revolving restaurant at its top; call (512) 299-8615.

As part of San Antonio's rejuvenation, the riverfront has been restored as a promenade, with boats, terraces, and cafes replacing rundown warehouses.

Event: Frontier Days
When: Last week in July
Where: Cheyenne, Wyoming

Contact: Cheyenne Frontier Days
P.O. Box 2666
Cheyenne, WY 82003
(307) 778-7200

Something about the event: This frontier festival sports one of the nation's largest outdoor rodeos. There are parades, chuck-wagon races, and an art show.

Accommodations with a personal touch:

Two Bars Seven Ranch (R), Box 67G, Tie Siding, WY 82084, (307) 742-6072: 14 rms, 10 pb, $52 ($15 each additional person); cc-no; c-yes, s-ltd, d-ltd, p-ltd, Full Bkfst; h-Polly Schaffer. This 8,000-acre cattle ranch along the Wyoming–Colorado border has been in the same family since it was built in 1860.

Bed and Breakfast Rocky Mountains (S), P.O. Box 804, Colorado Springs, CO 80901, (303) 630-3433

Roadside food: Hickory House, 11th and Logan, (307) 638-1445, is a cowboy hangout that serves hickory-smoked beef brisket, beans, and Polish sausages. At **Little America,** 2800 West Lincoln Way, Cheyenne, (307) 634-2771, a major tourist stop, there's a daily buffet that offers specialties from different lands—one day French, the next Greek, and so on. The crowd is often as entertaining as the meal. The **Whipple House,** 300 East 17th Street, (307) 634-2771, features game dishes served up in American and continental entrees. The **Hitching Post Inn,** 1700 Lincoln Way, (307) 638-3301, has won awards for its gourmet dishes, including chicken sesame, fish, and beef.

Some readings to enhance travels: Larson, Taft A., *Wyoming,* Norton, 1977; Hutton, Harold, *Vigilante Days: Frontier Justice along the Niobara,* Ohio University Press, 1978; Sodaro, Craig, and Adams, Rocky, *The Frontier Spirit: The Story of Wyoming,* Johnson, 1986.

Bakken, Larry, *Justice in the Wilderness: A Study of the Frontier Courts in Canada and the United States 1670–1870,* Rothman, 1986; Branch, E. Douglas, *The Cowboy and His Interpreter* (reprint of 1926 ed.), Applebaum, 1968; Cook, James H., *Fifty Years on the Old Frontier as Cowboy, Guide, Scout and Ranchman,* University of Oklahoma Press, 1981; Leyborn, James G., *Frontier Folkways,* Shoe String, 1970.

Turn off here along the way: The wild times of the Frontier Days in Cheyenne recall the real thing in the mid- to late 1860s, when the town was a frontier outpost full of speculators, gamblers, and real estate sharks. So notorious was Cheyenne's reputation that it was nicknamed "Hell on Wheels." In 1869 it became the capital of Wyoming.

The **Old West Museum,** North Carey Avenue, next to Frontier Park, (307) 778-7291, chronicles the history of the area and features horse-drawn vehicles and Indian artifacts. A special exhibit describes the impact of the Union Pacific Railroad on the region.

Speaking of the rails, **"Big Boy"** is one of the world's largest steam engines. It's not in use any more, but can be seen at Holliday Park.

Cheyenne's capitol building dominates its more conventional neighbors. Inside it is decorated with marble and murals. Tours are available; call (307) 777-7220. Nearby, in the Barrett Building at 24th and Central, (307) 777-7024, is the **State Museum.**

The **National First Day Cover Museum,** 702 Randall Avenue, (307) 634-5911, exhibits first day stamp covers of all kinds, from historical to scientific. Philatelic art is also on display.

A bit of the Old West can still be seen at **Wyoming Hereford Farm,** five miles east of Cheyenne on I-80, (307) 634-1905, a working cattle operation open to the public.

Event: State Fair (Colorado)
When: Last week in August through Labor Day
Where: Pueblo, Colorado

Contact: Colorado State Fair
Fairgrounds
Pueblo, CO 81004
(719) 561-8484

Something about the event: The state fair offers 11 days of midway fun, rides, entertainment, and a first-class rodeo. There is a special Mexican day.

Accommodations with a personal touch:
The **Hearthstone Inn** (I), 586 North Cascade Avenue, Colorado Springs, CO 80903, (719) 473-4413: 23 rms, pb, $55-90; cc-AE, MC, V; c-yes, s-ltd, d-no, p-no, Full Bkfst. Queen Victoria mansion from 1855, decorated in Victorian fashion, with 124 windows.

Bed and Breakfast Rocky Mountains (S), P.O. Box 804, Colorado Springs, CO 80901, (303) 630-3433.

Roadside food: Two local Mexican favorites are **Papa Felipe's,** 3297 Dillon Drive, (719) 542-1648, and **Natchos Fireside,** 801 Highway 50W, (719) 542-4557, where the specialty is a giant burrito that can feed two. **La Renaissance,** 217 East Routt, (719) 543-6367, is noteworthy for steaks, fish, and chicken served in a remodeled old church turned restaurant.

Some readings to enhance travels: Bryan, Ray, *Four Historic Walking Tours of Pueblo, Colorado,* Pueblo County Historical Society, 1983; Bancroft, Caroline, *Colorful Colorado, Its Dramatic History,* Johnson, 1959; Dallas, Sandra, *Colorado Ghost Towns and Mining Camps,* University of Oklahoma Press, 1985; May, Stephen, *Pilgrimage: A Journey through Colorado's History and Culture,* Ohio University Press, 1986.

Neely, Wayne C., *Agricultural Fair,* AMS Press (reprint of 1935 ed.), 1981; Schramm, Henry W., *The New York State Fair: An Empire Showcase,* North Country, 1985; Primmack, Phil, *New England Country Fair,* Globe Pequot, 1985; Walford, Cornelius, *Fairs Past and Present, A Chapter in the History of Commerce,* B. Franklin, 1967; Woolston, Bill, *Iowa's Fair,* Thorn Creek Press, 1975.

Turn off here along the way: Pueblo, located to the east of the Front Range of the Rocky Mountains at the confluence of the Arkansas River and Fountain Creek, was a regional center during the area's mining days, when the population multiplied eight times over in just ten years.

Today Pueblo is a Hispanic town. The area's history, especially the impact of iron and steel, is on display at **El Pueblo Museum,** 905 South Prairie Avenue, (719) 564-5274.

To the north, on I-25, is Colorado Springs, an agreeable city that is home to the **U.S. Air Force Academy,** 12 miles north of town on I-25, (719) 472-2553.

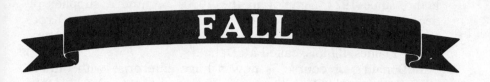

FALL

The Original Spuds

Officials in Boise, Idaho, do not push the potato. The state is trying to diversify, they say. Diversified or not, people still do not associate Idaho with computers or plastics. But the baked potato—now, that's Idaho.

The potato is a most American crop. In fact, it was growing in the New World before the New World was discovered. The 16th-century explorer Francisco Pizarro brought it back to Spain from Peru. It made its way back across the Atlantic in 1719, when Irish potato farmers settled in Londonderry, New Hampshire. Today, the potato is produced in more than 130 countries.

Potato growers like to remind anyone who will listen that their product, without butter, contains only 75 to 100 calories. Potatoes contain 75 percent water and are long on fiber and Vitamin C. But some people find it hard to consider potatoes a "nutritious food," since they're best known as a greasy accompaniment to "fast food" burgers.

Believe it or not, some 400 million hundredweight (100-pound sacks) of potatoes were produced in 1987, according to the Department of Agriculture. Of this total, 192 million were processed into 97 million french fries and 45 million potato chips.

The potato chip was "invented," so the story goes, in 1853 in Saratoga Springs, New York. A short-order (and short-tempered) cook, reacting to criticism of his culinary prowess, sought revenge by slicing potatoes thin and placing them in a deep fryer. The result of his rage was soon all the rage.

French fries, on the other hand, were introduced to the United States by President Thomas Jefferson, a Francophile, who first served them at the White House. But it was J. R. Simplot who put the french fry on the map. A farmer and rancher in Caldwell,

Idaho, since 1924, Simplot in the 1950s became a supplier of dehydrated frozen potatoes to a businessman named Ray Kroc, who served them alongside his hamburgers at a roadside eatery in Des Plaines, Illinois, called McDonald's.

McDonald's, of course, is now a huge enterprise with outlets all over the world. And its success is shared by Simplot's, potato supplier to the Golden Arches. In 1988, the number of potatoes processed into french fries at Simplot's ran into the billions.

How does a potato become a french fry? Fred Zersa, who works for Simplot's, explains that potatoes are harvested in the fall and are taken directly to the plant for processing or to a refrigerated storage facility, where they may be kept for up to a year to ensure a steady supply. At the plant, the potatoes are washed, steam-peeled, and sorted to eliminate those with defects. Each process is performed by machine.

Next comes the cutting process. But here matters are not quite as simple, for Simplot's produces one hundred different cuts of french fries. "Except for our biggest sellers," says Zersa, "we interchange the blades on the cutting instruments to account for the various specialty fries."

Once the cutting is completed, the slices are sorted by computer photography. "It's a computer defect-detection system that isolates the bad potatoes through pictures," says Zersa. "Then a knife-like device removes the defective potatoes."

The 30-minute production process ends with blanching, in which potatoes are partially cooked in oil, then quick-frozen for distribution.

They had better freeze well. These potatoes may travel not only to New York or Los Angeles, but as far away as Japan and Europe.

Some fifteen hundred people work on potato processing at the Caldwell plant, helping to process one hundred thousand pounds of raw potatoes per hour, 24 hours a day.

Shelley, Idaho, is a place where folks take the time to celebrate the potato once each year with games, music, and crafts as part of Idaho Spud Day (see page 159). They crown a Miss Russett, who presides over a breakfast featuring—you guessed it—hash brown potatoes. Then she leads the Spud Day Parade to the park, where a free baked potato is given to every participant.

Later that afternoon is held the World Championship Spud Picking Contest. Although the farms in the area are mechanized, here the picking is done by hand, the old-fashioned way, with contestants required to transfer loose potatoes by basket into large burlap bags. Whoever fills the bags first is declared champion and wins a trophy.

Although the potato does not receive the acclaim of more glamorous products, like oranges in Florida or lobsters in Maine, someday folks may come to appreciate it. In the meantime, in Idaho, the potato prevails.

Event: Idaho Spud Day
When: Third Saturday in September
Where: Shelley, Idaho

Contact: Chamber of Commerce
P.O. Box 301
Shelley, Idaho 83274
(208) 357-3457

Something about the event: The region celebrates its native crop with parades, games, music, and the World Championship Spud Picking Contest. Everyone gets a free baked potato.

Accommodations with a personal touch:
Pension Hermine (I), 937 West 200 South, Blackfoot, ID 83221, (208) 684-3857: 3 rms, pb-no, $25-35; cc-no; c-yes, s-yes, d-no, p-ltd, Full Bkfst; h-Hermine Balbi. Country pension in the midst of potato and grain fields. Approximately 30 minutes from Shelley.

Roadside food: Idaho boasts an eatery where potatoes are served up for dessert in the form of potato ice cream. This unique restaurant is **Reed's,** 2660 West Broadway, Idaho Falls, (208) 522-0123. The potato ice cream is lowfat and is produced in the dairy attached to the restaurant. Other features at Reed's include homemade soups served in bowls made from homemade breads.

Some readings to enhance travels: Conley, Curt, *Idaho for the Curious: A Guide,* Backeday, 1982; Federal Writers' Project, American Guide Series, *Idaho: A Guide in Word and Pictures,* Oxford University Press, 1950; Peterson, F. Ross, *Idaho,* Norton, 1977; Wells, Merle, and Hart, Arthur A., *Idaho: Gem of the Mountains,* Windsor, 1985.
Galvin, E. Michael, ed., *Potato World Handbook,* GDL, 1980; Hoge, Tom, *Potato Cookery,* Cornerstone, 1980; Turner, James H., *The Spud Book: 101 Ways to Cook Potatoes,* St. Martin's, 1982; Jones, Jeanne, *100 Meals in a Potato: Stuffed Spuds,* Evans, 1982.

Turn off here along the way: Shelley is situated along the Snake River on old U.S. Route 26, which runs parallel to I-15. To the northeast, near a cataract in the river, is **Idaho Falls,** a regional cultural center with a large Mormon population.

In the other direction, Fort Hall and Pocatello sit on lands that once belonged to the Fort Hall Indian Reservation. Pocatello was founded as a railway town and today is home to **Idaho State University.**

Event: Republic of Texas Chilympiad
When: Third weekend in September
Where: San Marcos, Texas

Contact: Republic of Texas Chilympiad
P.O. Box 188
San Marcos, TX 78666
(512) 396-5400

Something about the event: A major event in the world of chili, this cook-off tests top chefs in the home of the hot stuff.

Accommodations with a personal touch:
   Aquarena Springs Inn (I), Aquarena Drive, P.O. Box 2330, San Marcos, TX 78666, (512) 396-8901: 24 rms, pb, $50-65; cc-AE, DC, DISC, MC, V; c-yes, s-yes, d-no, p-no, Cont Bkfst; h-Paul Trottman. Old-fashioned, high-ceilinged inn in midst of Aquarena Park. Olympic-size and smaller-size swimming pools.
   Crystal River Inn (B&B), 326 West Hopkins, San Marcos, TX 78666, (512) 396-3739: 8 rms, 6 pb, $45-65; cc-MC, V; c-no, s-no, d-yes, p-no, Full Bkfst; h-Kathy Dillon. Restored Victorian inn with fireplaces, courtyards, and sitting rooms.
   Bed and Breakfast of Wimberly, Texas (S), P.O. Box 589, Wimberly, TX 78676, (512) 847-9666.

Roadside food: Palmer's Restaurant, Ranch Road 12 and Hutchinson, San Marcos, (512) 353-3500, features more than 100 items on the menu, including charbroiled steak and broccoli cheese soup. Barbecue is the specialty at the **Guadaloupe Smoked Meat Co.,** Green Road, New Braunfels, (512) 629-6121. Surprisingly, there is not much to recommend in chili in the area; there's enough of that at the cook-off anyway.

Some readings to enhance travels: Butel, Jane, *Chili Madness,* Workman, 1980; Fischer, Mildred and Al, *Chili Lovers' Cookbook,* Golden West, 1978; Griffith, Dotty, *Wild about Chili,* Barron, 1985;

Wagner, Candy, and Marquez, Sandra, *Cooking Texas Style: A Heritage of Traditional Recipes,* University of Texas Press, 1983. See also "Texas Folklife Festival," page 152.

Turn off here along the way: San Marcos developed around the springs emerging from a geological fault line. The location has been turned into an entertainment area featuring boat rides and underwater shows in a "Submarine Theater." The grounds include an inn and an 18th-century Spanish mission. The highlight at the park is a diving pig.

San Marcos stands near I-35 halfway between Austin and San Antonio. The area is heavily influenced by Hispanic culture, but many other ethnicities play a part as well. German influence may be seen in **New Braunfels,** first settled in 1845. The town still maintains a German connection through its architecture and culture. See also page 167.

Event: Bison Roundup
When: First week in October
Where: Moiese, Montana

Contact: Refuge Manager
National Bison Range
Moiese, Montana 59824
(406) 644-2211

Something about the event: Some 300 to 500 bison range over 19,000 acres of grassland and timber on the National Bison Range. The autumn roundup is open for public viewing.

Accommodations with a personal touch:
  Western Bed and Breakfast Hosts (S), P.O. Box 322, Kalispell, MT 59901, (406) 257-4476.

Roadside food: Quite a few restaurants feature the likes of bison burgers, buffalo stew, and buffalo steaks, all of which are said to taste sweeter than their beef counterparts. Restaurants serving up these specialties include **Wrangler Restaurant,** 302 Mount Rushmore Road, (605) 673-4271, and **Sylvan Lake Lodge,** in the park, Highway 87/89, Hill City, (605) 574-2561.

Some readings to enhance travels: Malone, Michael P., *Montana: A History of Two Centuries,* University of Washington Press, 1977;

Spence, Clark C., *Montana,* Norton, 1978; Federal Writers' Project, American Guide Series, *Montana: A State Guide Book,* Viking, 1939.

Allen, Joel, *The American Bisons Living and Extinct,* Ayer, 1974; Garretson, Marli, *A Short History of the American Bison,* Ayer, (reprint of 1934 ed.); Patent, Dorothy H., *Buffalo: The American Bison Today,* Ticknor & Fields, 1986; Sample, Michael S., *Bison: Symbol of the American West,* Falcon, 1987; Sandoz, Mari, *The Buffalo Hunters: The Story of the Hide Men,* University of Nebraska Press, 1978.

Turn off here along the way: In addition to buffalo, the **National Bison Range** is home to elk, deer, and antelope. Tours are available, but there are restrictions. For particulars, stop at the Visitors Center at the Moiese entrance or call (406) 644-2211.

Southeast along U.S. 93, the region's main north–south thoroughfare, **St. Ignatius** is the site of a mission built in 1854. A dry fresco executed by a mission cook at the turn of the century adorns the church's interior.

Polson, also along U.S. 93, is a community at the foot of Flathead Lake. According to some local folks, the legendary Paul Bunyan dug the channel that connects the Flathead River with Flathead Lake.

Event: Norsfest and Lutefisk Day
When: Second weekend in November
Where: Madison, Minnesota

Contact: Lutefisk Day
c/o Dick Jackson
Super Valu
208 Seventh Avenue
Madison, MN 56256
(612) 598-7448

Something about the event: Lutefisk is codfish boiled, soaked in lye, and covered with lard drippings. The Minnesota towns of Madison and Glenwood have an ongoing feud over which one is the true lutefisk capital. Glenwood holds its festival in May. Madison's, in November, includes a dinner with "the Wild Norwegian," arts, crafts, and other festivities to celebrate the "delicacy" that Norwegians love to hate.

Accommodations with a personal touch:
Bed and Breakfast Upper Midwest (S), P.O. Box 28036, Crystal Lake, MN 55428, (612) 535-7135.
Bed and Breakfast Registry (S), P.O. Box 8174, St. Paul, MN 55108, (612) 646-4238.

Roadside food: Madison is one of the few places where lutefisk can actually be found in a restaurant. The place is the **North Forty Cafe,** 317 Sixth Avenue, (612) 598-7497, where the food is Norwegian. For less daring souls, the **Pantry Cafe,** 217 Sixth Avenue, (612) 598-3377, serves traditional American home-style food.

Some readings to enhance travels: Gjerde, Jon, *From Peasants to Farmers: The Migration from Balestrand, Norway, to the Upper Midwest,* Cambridge University Press, 1985; Qualey, Carlton C., *Norwegian Settlement in the United States,* Ayer, 1970 (reprint of 1938 ed.); Roalson, Louise, *Notably Norwegian: Recipes, Festivals, Folk Arts,* Penfield, 1982; Scott, Astrid K., *Ekte Norsk Mat (Authentic Norwegian Cooking),* Graphic, 1983. See also "Festival of Nations," page 144.

Turn off here along the way: Madison lies in western Minnesota, in Lac Qui Parle County, a region that was first settled by the French. The lands became American as part of the Louisiana Purchase. Today the area is agricultural. The nearby city of **Granite Falls** has a hydroelectric power plant on the Minnesota River.

Hanley Falls is an old railroad town that took the railroads to the U.S. Supreme Court to force them to allow passengers to transfer from one line to another. The **Yellow Medicine Agricultural and Transportation Museum,** two blocks north of the junction of S.R. 23 and C.R. 18, (507) 768-3522, displays farm machinery and artifacts.

Event: Will Rogers Day
When: November (Rogers's birthday is November 4)
Where: Claremore, Oklahoma

Contact: Chamber of Commerce
P.O. Box 984
Claremore, OK 74018
(918) 341-2818

Something about the event: Will Rogers's home is the location for an annual birthday celebration in honor of the humorist. Activities include a parade, arts and crafts, a chili cook-off, and a humor-writing contest.

Accommodations with a personal touch:
  Country Inn Bed and Breakfast (B&B), Route 3, Box 1925, Claremore, OK 74017, (918) 342-1894: 2 rms, pb, $30-35; cc-no; c-no, s-no, d-no, p-no, Full Bkfst; h-Leland Jenkins. Barn-style B&B located in Oklahoma "Green Country" 15 minutes northeast of Claremore.
  Will Rogers Hotel (H), 524 West Will Rogers Boulevard, Claremore, OK 74017, (918) 341-0861: 50 rms, 5 pb, $17.50-$45; cc-MC, V; c-ltd, s-yes, d-yes, p-no, Bkfst-no. Restored hotel. Old-time ambience and famous mineral baths.

Roadside food: Think of Oklahoma, and your mouth will start to water from thoughts of barbecue, fried chicken, and other regional specialties. All may be found around Claremore. Oklahoma-style barbecue is served up at **Cotton Eye Joe's,** 715 Morentz, (918) 342-0855. **Dot's Cafe,** 310 West Will Rogers Boulevard, (918) 341-9718, features chicken-fried steak and fried chicken. The **Golden Corral Restaurant,** 1405 West Will Rogers Boulevard, (918) 342-5510, offers steak in a family-style atmosphere.

Some readings to enhance travels: Bennett, Cathleen L., *Will Rogers: The Cowboy Who Walked with Kings,* Ameron; Graught, Steven K., *He Chews To Run: Will Rogers' Life Magazine Articles,* Oklahoma State University Press, 1982; Milstein, David, *Will Rogers: An Appreciation,* Gordon Press, 1976. See also "89er Days," page 145.

Turn off here along the way: In addition to being Will Rogers's hometown, Claremore is famous for its springs. It is a resort town where people come to ease their arthritis, rheumatism, and other ailments. There is also what is described as the largest gun collection in the world—20,000 items—at the **Davis Gun Museum,** Fifth and Lynn Riggs Boulevard, (918) 341-5707.

WINTER

One Good Bowl of the Hot Stuff

Few things are more southwestern than a good bowl of chili. The image is a familiar one—a husky man seated beside a bowl of "the hot stuff" with some onions, crackers, and a cold beer nearby. It seems so simple. But the world of chili is much more complex.

Few subjects raise passions as much as the question of how a good bowl of chili is made. In fact, the debate is often as hot as the chili peppers used to prepare the dish, which has often been described as "the people's food" because it transcends any formal school of cooking technique. Folks cannot even agree on what chili is or on how to spell it.

One thing is certain: Chili contains chili peppers, the fruit of capsicum plants. In New Mexico, both the dish and the pod are spelled *chile* (following the Spanish usage); elsewhere, both are spelled *chili;* and there are places where they are spelled *chilli.*

Chile in its traditional form is revered in New Mexico, where enthusiasts of the pepper go to great lengths to distance themselves from what they consider its misuse in the form of chili stew. A common sight along the roads of New Mexico is chile pods hanging out to dry on long chains called *ristres.* Through the fall and winter, and especially during Christmas, chiles are used not only for culinary purposes but for decoration as well.

Residents of New Mexico regard the chile pepper with more than a passing interest. They've formed the International Connoisseurs of Red and Green Chile, based in Las Cruces. The group's stated purpose is to clarify the distinction between pure chile and "the other stuff." They also devote their efforts to explaining the differences between red and green chiles and to describing their various uses. Through books, television programs, and classes they're out

167

to tell the world of the diversity of chiles. There's even a chile outreach program.

The group also encourages research on chiles. A research lab is housed at the University of New Mexico. It is an outgrowth of the first formal chile research performed there in 1907, when a professor set out to improve chile breeding capabilities.

Chili is said to have originated when poor Mexican families in Texas mixed chopped peppers into their meat in order to make it stretch farther. The dish gained prominence when vendors, known as chili queens, began dishing it up on the streets of San Antonio. They could be found there until the 1940s. The Texas phenomenon went national at the Chicago World's Fair of 1893, where San Antonio chili queens served a combination of chili and blended spices.

There are virtually thousands of different ways of making chili. To the traditional purist, chili means meat—not chopped meat, but cubes of lean beef—cooked with hot peppers. Anything else is not authentic. Modern-day chili purists often include tomatoes and kidney beans in their potions, along with such items as onions, garlic, and cumin. Secret ingredients may include beer, wine, Worcestershire sauce, or Dijon mustard.

As the popularity of chili increases, the number of variations grows. In California, one favorite recipe contains more vegetables and less meat. Wheat acts as a meat substitute in Veggie Chili, which may also include corn, zucchini, or olives. "Son-of-a-Gun Chili" contains organ meat—brains, heart, and liver—as well as muscle meat. It is reputed to have been a cowboy favorite. Three-hundred to 500 barrels of chili are served at the "Western Stock Show" in Denver (see page 169).

Although Texas and the Southwest are generally considered the home of chili, other regions have developed their own chili fetishes. One is Springfield, Illinois, which claims the title of Chilli Capital of the World. Chilli is thought to come to Springfield by way of the 1904 St. Louis World's Fair. At Springfield's Den Chilli Parlor, the chilli consists of peppers, kidney beans, and meat, and is available at five levels of intensity ranging from "mild" to "fire."

In Cincinnati, the local version is called Five Way Chili. It has seasoned ground meat, beans, spaghetti, onions, and cheese. Local legend has it that Cincinnati chili was discovered by Antl Kiradjieff, a Greek immigrant who arrived in the Queen City by way of New York, bringing with him hot dogs and chili dogs from Nathan's Famous in Coney Island. The chili hot dog endures in Cincinnati, and with the later addition of grated cheese, has become known locally as the Cheese Coney.

Larry Blundred of Skyline Chili in Cincinnati says their local chili "won't burn your insides like the Texas version." He describes it as "savory spicy," as opposed to the "hot dominant" found elsewhere in the land. "Some might call it slightly sweet," says Blundred.

Texans like to cast a disparaging eye at Cincinnati chili, but in fact many Southwest eateries offer a concoction called chili-mac—macaroni and cheese with chili. Indeed, culinary customs migrate so easily in contemporary America that chili hybrids are quite common.

Chili parlors of note may now be found in New England, New York City, California, and Oklahoma. After many years as an uncouth cousin, chili is now chic. (For more on chili, see the "Republic of Texas Chilympiad," page 160.)

Event: Western Stock Show
When: Mid-January
Where: Denver, Colorado

Contact: National Western Stock Show and Rodeo
1325 East 46th Avenue
Denver, CO 80216
(303) 295-1660

Something about the event: This is a major rodeo with more than 1,000 participants. There are also shows for horses, sheep, and 20 breeds of cattle. They serve some 300 to 500 barrels of homemade chili—ingredients include chili powder, cayenne, pinto beans, and ketchup. BBQ Beef, baked beans, and chicken fried steaks also available in abundance.

Accommodations with a personal touch:
The **Dove Inn** (I), 711 14th Street, Golden, CO 80401, (303) 278-2209: 6 rms, 4 pb, $36-54; cc-DC, MC, V; c-yes, s-no, d-no, p-no, Full Bkfst; h-Marylin Stephenson. Victorian inn from the 1880s, located minutes from Denver but away from the traffic and crowds. Special note on inn policy: no unmarried couples.

Oxford Hotel (H), 1600 17th Street, Denver, CO 80202, (303) 628-5400: 81 rms (10 suites), pb, $50-65; cc-AE, DISC, MC, V; c-yes, s-yes, d-no, p-no, Bkfst-no. Hotel, listed on National Register of Historic Places, dates back to 1891 and has been restored to look as it did then. Added feature is Art Deco bar.

The **Brown Palace** (H), 321 17th Street, Denver, CO 80202, (303) 297-3111: 250 rms, pb, $100-600; cc-AE, MC, V; c-yes, s-ltd, d-no, p-no, Bkfst-no. Denver's finest hotel, founded in 1892, features a "Casanova Room," Gold Room," and authentic restored period rooms.

Bed and Breakfast Colorado (S), P.O. Box 20596, Denver, CO 80220, (303) 333-3340.

Roadside food: Denver's come a long way from its days as a frontier cow town. But the atmosphere of those former days can be experienced at the **Buckhorn Exchange,** 1000 Osage Street, (303) 534-9505. It's a little out of the way, but well worth the trip. Dinner highlights are 24-ounce steaks and such unusual entrees as buffalo steaks and Rocky Mountain oysters (bulls' testicles). The dining room is furnished with trophies, antique guns, and an oak bar. Truly a restaurant with history. Also of note in town is **The Broker,** 821 17th Street, (303) 320-0757, which features steak and a complimentary one-and-a-half-pound shrimp bowl with dinner.

Some readings to enhance travels: Adams, Robert, *Denver: A Photographic Survey of the Metropolitan Area,* Colorado Association, 1977; Dorsett, Lyle, *The Queen City: A History of Denver,* Pruett, 1986; Morris, Langdon E., Jr., *Denver Landmarks,* C. W. Cleworth, 1979; Robinson, Linda, and Schneider, Vicki, *Mile High Denver: A Guide to the Queen City,* Pruett, 1981.

Cooper, Roy, *Calf Roping,* Western Horseman, 1984; Fleming, Steve, ed., *Official Professional Rodeo Guide,* Johnson, 1987; Frederickson, Kristine, *American Rodeo: From Buffalo Bill to Big Business,* Texas A&M Press, 1985; McGinnis, Carol, *Rodeo Days,* Ballantine, 1987; Ramirez, Nora, *The Southwestern Livestock Show and Rodeo,* Texas Western, 1972; Westermeier, Clifford M., *Man, Beast, Dust: The Story of Rodeo,* University of Nebraska Press, 1987.

Turn off here along the way: Denver gets one of its nicknames, Mile High City, from the altitude of the thirteenth step on the staircase of the **State Capitol,** Broadway and Colfax, (303) 866-4357. It is exactly 5,280 feet high. The dome of the capitol is covered with pure gold leaf.

Denver is also the home of the **U.S. Mint,** 320 West Colfax, (303) 844-3582. Tours are offered.

A unique museum environment is the **Denver Children's Museum,** 2121 Crescent Drive, (303) 433-7444. There are exhibits that teach through a hands-on experience. One is a grocery game. Another is a ball room with 80,000 balls.

The **Denver Art Museum,** at the Civic Center, 100 West 14th Street, (303) 575-2793, exhibits textiles and quilts. More than one million glass tiles were used in the building's construction. Art of the American West, including works by Bierstadt, Russell, Remington, and O'Keeffe, is on display at the **Museum of Western Art,** 1727 Tremont Place, (303) 296-1880.

The **Denver Center for the Performing Arts,** Champa and 14th Street, is home to theater and music, including the **Denver Symphony,** (303) 572-3046.

Event: Western Art Auction
When: Third weekend in March
Where: Great Falls, Montana

Contact: Great Falls Advertising Federation
P.O. Box 619
Great Falls, MT 59403
(406) 761-6453

Something about the event: Works of western art, past and present, are exhibited and auctioned at the Russell Museum. In addition, there are seminars and receptions. Held at C.M. Russell Museum which exhibits watercolors, sculptures, illustrations of great Western artists, all year long.

Accommodations with a personal touch:
Murphy's House Bed and Breakfast (B&B), 2020 Fifth Avenue North, Great Falls, MT 59401, (406) 452-3598: 2 rms, pb-no, $35-45; cc-no; c-no, s-yes, d-no, p-no, Full Bkfst; h-Mrs. H. T. Murphy. B&B six miles from the site of the auction.

Three Pheasant Inn (B&B), 626 Fifth Avenue North, Great Falls, MT 59401, (406) 453-0519: 4 rms, 1 pb, $32-45; cc-no; c-over 6, s-ltd, d-no, p-ltd, Full Bkfst; h-Amy and Dave Sloan. English Victorian antique-filled inn. Gazebo and fountain in private garden.

Western Bed and Breakfast Hosts (S), P.O. Box 322, Kalispell, MT 59901, (406) 257-4476.

Bed and Breakfast of the Rocky Mountains (S), P.O. Box 804, Colorado Springs, CO 80901, (303) 680-3433.

Roadside food: Beef and lamb are the foundation of the regional cuisine. **Eddie's Supper Club,** 3725 Second Avenue, Great Falls, (406) 453-1616, serves up a 22-ounce steak with baked potato. At **Borrie's,** 1800 Smelter Avenue, Black Eagle, (406) 761-0300, the T-bone steaks are said to roll over the sides of the platter.

Some readings to enhance travels: Yuill, Eilan R., *A Centennial Celebration: A History of Great Falls, Montana,* Yuill Enterprises, 1984.

Paladin, Vivian, ed., *C. M. Russell: The McKay Collection,* Montana Historical Society; Paladin, Vivian A., *Rendezvous of Western Art,* Montana Historical Society, 1975; Russell, Charles, *Paper Talk: Charlie Russell's Western Art,* Knopf, 1979; Harmen, Dorothy, *American Western Art,* M. Harmsen, 1978; Tyler, Ron, *American Frontier Life: Early Western Painting and Prints,* Abbeville Press, 1987. See also "Bison Roundup," page 161.

Turn off here along the way: Great Falls is situated in the Rockies, and the scenery is primarily what draws people to the area. It is the site of **Giant Springs,** the largest freshwater spring in the world. A collection of operable antique steam engines is on display at the **Mehmile Steam Museum** on U.S. 87-89, 10 miles east of Great Falls, (406) 452-6571.

To the south, along I-15, you will pass the scenic **Gates of the Mountain Wilderness.**

Further south is the state capital, **Helena,** founded at the site of a gold strike (on what is now Main Street).

Maysville, 25 miles to the northwest of Helena, is an authentic ghost town, a relic of the gold boom of the 1890s.

Event: Southwest Exposition
Fat Stock Show and Rodeo
When: Last weekend in January
through first weekend in February
Where: Fort Worth, Texas

Contact: Southwest Exposition Fat Stock Show and Rodeo
P.O. Box 150
Fort Worth, TX 76101
(817) 332-7361
(817) 877-2400

Something about the event: This event started in 1917 as the first indoor rodeo. Today, it also features livestock displays, horse shows, a midway, western food, and entertainment. Texas chili is among the foods served at the show.

Accommodations with a personal touch:
Stockyards Hotel (H), P.O. Box 4558, Fort Worth, TX 76106,

(817) 625-6427: 52 rms, pb, $89-350; cc-AE, DC, MC, V; c-yes, s-yes, d-yes, p-no, Bkfst-no. Landmark hotel in Fort Worth's Stockyards District, restored with modern conveniences.

Melrose Hotel (H), 3015 Oaklawn Avenue, Dallas, TX 75219, (214) 521-5151: 185 rms, pb, $79-195; cc-AE, CB, DC, MC, V; c-yes, s-yes, d-yes, p-ltd, Bkfst-no. Restored landmark hotel, reopened in 1985, features marble-floored lobby, Art Deco dining room, and English country library-style bar.

Hotel Crescent Court (H), 400 Crescent Court, Dallas, TX 75201, (214) 871-3200: 218 rms, pb, $180-350; cc-AE, DISC, MC, V; c-yes, s-yes, d-ltd, p-yes, Bkfst-no. This 19th-century hotel, rebuilt in 1985, retains its oversize windows and luxurious rooms and food.

Bed and Breakfast Texas Style (S), 4224 West Red Bird Lane, Dallas, TX 75237, (214) 298-8596.

Roadside food: Williams Ranch House, 5532 Jacks Boro, (817) 624-1272, has been a family restaurant for more than 30 years. It features barbecue and steak. **Massey's,** 1805 Eighth Avenue, (817) 924-8242, is the home of the chicken-fried steak. It comes with heaps of gravy and biscuits. **Star Cafe,** 111 West Exchange, (817) 624-8701, offers steaks grilled with butter and half-pound burgers, along with chicken-fried steak.

Some readings to enhance travels: Williams, Mack H., *In Old Fort Worth*, Williams, 1977. For books on Texas, see "Texas Folklife Festival," page 152. For books on rodeo, see "Western Stock Show," page 170.

Turn off here along the way: Once a cow town, Fort Worth, known as "The Most Texan of Texas Cities," has maintained its frontier flavor. It stands in sharp contrast to the futuristic Dallas–Fort Worth Airport and the skyscrapers of downtown Dallas. The historic **Stockyards District** has been cleaned up and restored; mechanized yards now process livestock. Four universities call Fort Worth home. There are many art museums, as well as ballet, opera, and concerts. Restaurants, galleries, and crafts shops are found at **Sundance Square,** near Main Street.

Event: Basque Sheepherders' Ball and Lamb Auction
When: Last weekend in January
Where: Boise, Idaho

Contact: Basque Center
601 Grove
Boise, ID 83701
(208) 342-9983

Something about the event: The Basques came to North America from the Pyrenees Mountains in France and Spain, where they were sheepherders. In America, many took up the same occupation in the mountains of the West. In the summer, they meet at the Basque Festival in Nevada; in the winter, they gather in Idaho to celebrate their language, foods, music, and cultural heritage.

Accommodations with a personal touch:
   Idaho City Hotel (H), P.O. Box 70, Idaho City, ID 83631, (208) 392-4290: 5 rms, pb, $26-36; cc-AE, MC, V; c-yes, s-yes, d-no, p-yes, Full Bkfst; h-Doc Campbell. Old West hotel, furnished with antiques, was built by Chinese in Idaho City's Chinatown. Rare Chinese coins were recently unearthed from its backyard. A 45-minute drive from Boise.
   Northwest Bed and Breakfast (S), 7707 Southwest Locust Street, Portland, OR 97231, (503) 746-8366.

Roadside food: A recent addition to the restaurant scene in Boise is **Onati,** 620 West Idaho, (208) 343-6464. The cuisine is Basque, highlighted by lamb and sweetbread.

Some readings to enhance travels: Douglass, William A., *Basque Sheepherders of the American West: A Photographic Documentary,* University of Nevada Press, 1985; Errecart, Felipa M., *Hang Tough! Basque Cooking, Life and Ways,* Strawberry Hill, 1988; Ott, Sandra, *The Circle of Mountains: A Basque Sheepherding Community,* Oxford University Press, 1981. See also "Idaho Spud Day," page 159.

Turn off here along the way: Some of Boise's summer attractions remain open in the winter. The **State Capitol,** Jefferson and West State between 6th and 8th Streets, (208) 334-2411, is a sandstone structure that took 15 years to complete. A gold eagle perches on its top; within is a statue of George Washington.

Other indoor attractions include the **Boise Art Museum,** 670 South Julia Davis Drive, (208) 345-8330, and the **Idaho Historical Society Museum,** 610 North Julia Davis Drive, (208) 334-2120, which contains a Chinese temple and 19th-century buildings from early Idaho.

But the real beauty is outdoors. The **Boise National Forest** is in an area of abandoned mining towns and shafts where elk, deer, and other wildlife wander. Cross-country skiing is available. For information, contact the Forest Visitors Center at 1750 Front Street, (208) 334-1516.

To the north of Boise is Idaho City, the largest city in the West in 1862. Many period buildings still stand. The era is recalled at the **Idaho City Museum,** Montgomery Street at Wall Street, (208) 392-4550.

Event: St. Paul Winter Carnival
When: Last weekend in January
through the first weekend of February
Where: St. Paul, Minnesota

Contact: St. Paul Winter Carnival
339 Bremer Building
St. Paul, MN 55101
(612) 222-4416

Something about the event: The carnival was started in 1886. Today, there are more than 100 events, both indoors and outdoors, over the course of the ten-day celebration. Highlights include a sleigh and cutter parade that recreates Currier and Ives scenes, winter sports competitions, music and art, ice sculptures, and a grand parade that draws up to 75,000

Accommodations with a personal touch: See "Festival of Nations," page 143.

Roadside food: See "Festival of Nations," page 143.

Some readings to enhance travels: For books on Minnesota and St. Paul, see "Festival of Nations," page 144. For books on ice carving, see "Lakeside Winter Celebration," page 131.

Turn off here along the way: The Greater Twin Cities area is a mecca for the arts, shopping, and sightseeing. When you have finished gazing at those beautiful ice sculptures in Landmark Square, you might go to warm up in **Landmark Center,** 75 West Fifth Street, (612) 292-3225. Originally a federal court building modeled after Boston's Trinity Church, it was built completely with local materials and is replete with wood paneling, stained glass, and fireplaces. Today the building houses a branch of the **Minnesota Museum of Art,** the **Shubert Piano Museum,** and many special events.

Another branch of the Museum of Art is located at Kellogg Boulevard and St. Peter Street, (612) 292-4355. Contemporary and Asian arts are featured.

Minneapolis, the Twin City on the west bank of the Mississippi, is a world-class city offering great diversity. On arriving, one first notices the booming downtown area. Downtown landmarks include the 57-story **IDS Tower** at 8th Street and Nicollet Avenue, which is the largest building between Chicago and San Francisco, and the **Hubert H. Humphrey Metrodome,** 900 South 5th Street, (662) 332-0386, an imposing domed stadium that is home to the Minnesota Twins (baseball) and Vikings (football). But downtown Minneapolis is best known for its comprehensive network of skyways (indoor walkways) that interconnect some 17 blocks of downtown offices and shopping malls and protect Minnesotans from their "brisk" winters.

Culture abounds in Minneapolis. **Orchestra Hall,** 1111 Nicollet Mall, (612) 371-5636, is home of the renowned Minnesota Orchestra and host to a variety of big-name entertainment. Music and drama are offered at the **Guthrie Theatre,** 725 Vineland Place, (612) 377-2224. In the same complex is the **Walker Arts Center,** (612) 375-7600, which has one of the country's premier collections of contemporary art. The Walker recently unveiled a new outdoor sculpture garden.

Minneapolis is also a city of outdoor beauty. Twenty-two lakes and 153 parks may be found within city limits. They draw active Minnesotans even in the coldest weather (the cross-country ski trails are busy even in −15 degree weather). For information about the parks and their activities, call (612) 348-PARK.

The St. Croix River, one of America's designated wild and scenic rivers, merges with the Mississippi just south of St. Paul. A number of scenic, historic Mississippi River towns are nearby. Side trips to Taylors Falls, Stillwater, Hastings, and Red Wing offer quaint inns, antique shops, and many restored buildings, as well as stores and galleries to stroll through.

Finally, a unique day outdoors may be had at **Amodt's Apple Farm and Cross-Country Ski Trails,** 6428 Manning Avenue North,

P.O. Box 295, Stillwater, MN 55028, (612) 439-3127. There, an apple orchard is transformed into a winter wonderland. Cross-country skiers can pass among 6,000 apple trees and evergreens. Nonskiers can enjoy horsedrawn sleigh rides. Afterward, there is cider and hot apple pie and soup served up in an old barn and farmhouse with a pot-bellied stove.

See also "Festival of Nations," page 143.

WEST

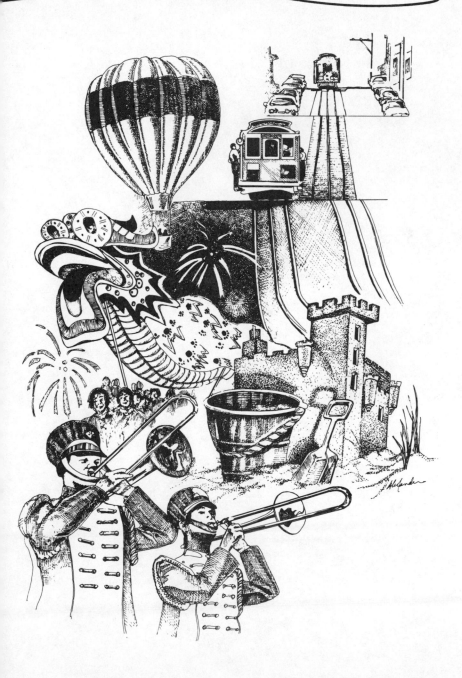

SPRING

Neighbors on the Border

Spanish-American culture is at once native and foreign. Spanish was spoken here centuries before there was a United States. Today, the prevalence of Hispanic culture along the southern border of the United States is celebrated by some and deplored by others, depending on the political and social winds of the day.

The United States–Mexico border is often profiled in the news as the site of illegal crossings, both of aliens and of drugs. However, the real story of the two-thousand-mile border between the two nations is the self-contained, mutually dependent nature of the region.

There are seven "sister cities" that straddle the border. The easternmost pair is Brownsville, Texas, and Matamoros, Tamaulipas, on the Gulf of Mexico. The westernmost pair is San Diego, California, and Tijuana, Baja, on the Pacific Ocean. All seven display symbiotic relationships similar to the one that exists between Nogales, Arizona, and Nogales, Sonora.

The two Nogaleses and their common border serve as the focal point for ongoing trade between the two nations. Fruits and vegetables from Mexico pass through Arizona on their way north for distribution in the United States and Canada, while American goods (appliances, technology, and tourists) go through in the other direction. At the same time, factories have been built on both sides of the border to take advantage of the enormous labor force (more than 7 million people live along the border, and another 14 million live within one hundred miles of it).

"It's a blend of American, Mexican-American, and Mexican national cultures," says John A. Garcia, professor of Latin American Studies at the University of Arizona. "There's this continual

181

crossover—things like language, where you can frequently hear a sentence started in English and finished in Spanish."

The region was used as a smuggling route as far back as the 1700s. In 1880, word spread that the Southern Pacific Railroad line would be built through Nogales Pass. Jacob Issaacson, an itinerant merchant, set up an inn, anticipating business when the train arrived. A Mexican custom house was also established. Soon Issaactown—renamed Nogales because of the many Walnut trees (*nogal* in Spanish)—became a thriving community.

Susan Spater of the Pimeria Alta Historical Society points out that between 1880 and 1916 not even a fence separated Nogales, Mexico, and Nogales, U.S.A. The towns are separated today by International Avenue with a wall and customs. The Ambos Nogales Commission, whose slogan reads "One Great City—Two Great Countries," explores ways of improving the local economy, tourist trade, agriculture, and industry.

The history and cultural unity shared by the two Nogaleses is publicly celebrated on Cinco de Mayo, the Fifth of May (see "Cinco de Mayo," page 183). Many Americans believe that Cinco de Mayo is Mexican Independence Day. In fact, it marks an important victory for Mexican forces over Napoleon's invading French troops in 1862.

The day is celebrated throughout Mexico. In addition, the festivities spill over into Arizona, New Mexico, Texas, and California, where fiestas, music, dancing, Mexican food, and general merriment prevail. The cornerstone of the celebration is the *pinada*, a clay pot decorated with bright tissue paper and hung from the ceiling. When it's broken, candy and toys fall into the hands of waiting children.

In Nogales, the celebration takes place on both sides of the border. Families are reunited in a party that lasts well into the night. The highlight is the parade that crosses and re-crosses the border, taking hours as it weaves through the narrow streets of both Nogaleses.

Mexican Independence Day (September 16) and Christmas are also times of joint celebrations on both sides of the border. However, according to Susan Spater, these observances are not nearly as interesting as November 2, a Mexican holiday called the Day of the Dead, when families gather at the graves of loved ones. "It's reflective," says Spater, "but it's joyous and colorful as well."

The cultural and economic interdependence of Mexico and the United States extend beyond the border areas to the North. In Tucson, locals celebrate Mexican Independence with four days of celebration in Kennedy Park and Oury Park. The music is performed by many groups who travel north from Mexico to celebrate this most Mexican of holidays.

Each year in April, Tucson also plays host to a Mariachi Conference that attracts groups from throughout the United States and Mexico. One year, pop singer Linda Ronstadt, whose father is part Mexican, was featured as a special guest. (The Ronstadt name stretches back to 1888 in Tucson musical circles.) A long tradition of Spanish theater thrives in Tucson, too.

To Susan Spater, life in Nogales is not that different from Ames, Iowa. "It's local politics," she says. "It's just that our local issues are important to local residents who happen to be citizens and residents of two countries."

Event: Cinco de Mayo
When: May 1
Where: Nogales, Arizona

Contact: Chamber of Commerce
Kino Park
Nogales, AZ 85621
(602) 287-3685

Something about the event: International community along the Mexican-American border, commemorates the Mexican victory over France in a pivotal battle on May 5, 1862. Fiesta of music, dance, and Mexican food.

Accommodations with a personal touch:
  Arizona Inn (H), 200 East Elm Street, Tucson, AZ, (602) 325-1541: 85 rms, pb, $52-400; cc-MC, AE, V; c-yes, s-yes, d-yes, p-no, Full Bkfst. Southwestern architecture, circa 1930, and Old World charm on 14 acres. An oasis in Tucson.
  Hacienda del Sol (H), Hacienda del Sol Road, Tucson, AZ 85718, (602) 299-1501: 36 rms, 34 pb, $29-125; cc-MC, AE, V; c-yes, s-yes, d-yes, p-ltd, Cont Bkfst; h-Debby Whitney. Adobe inn from 1929, one of the last authentic southwestern buildings in the area.
  Bed and Breakfast in Arizona (S), 8433 North Black Canyon, Suite 150, Phoenix, AZ 85021, (602) 995-2831.
  Mi Casa Su Casa Bed and Breakfast (S), P.O. Box 950, Tempe, AZ 85281, (602) 990-0682.

Roadside food: Not surprisingly, when it comes to cuisine, all eyes look south. Two favorites in the Nogales across the border are **El**

Cid, Avenita Obregon 124, Tel. 264-00, which specializes in seafood and fowl, and **La Roca,** Calle Elias 91, Tel. 207-60, which serves both Mexican and American dishes.

Some readings to enhance travels: Powell, Lawrence C., *Arizona,* Norton, 1976; Lesure, Thomas B., *All about Arizona,* Harian, 1983; Trimble, Marshall, *Arizona: A Panoramic History of a Frontier State,* Doubleday, 1977; Federal Writers' Project, American Guide Series, *Arizona: The Grand Canyon State,* Hastings, 1980.

Basch, Samuel, *Memories of Mexico: History of the Last Ten Months of the Empire,* Trinity University Press, 1973; Dabbs, Jack, *The French Army in Mexico, 1861–1867: A Study in Military Government,* Mouton, 1963; Baird, Peter, and McCaughtan, Ed, eds., *Beyond the Border: Mexico and the U.S. Today,* Congress of Latin America, 1979, Gibson, Lay J., and Renteria, Alfonso C., *The U.S. and Mexico: Borderland Development and the National Economics,* Westview, 1985.

Turn off here along the way: In Nogales, the **Pimeria Alta Historical Society,** Old City Hall, (602) 287-5402, exhibits the history of the area. On the Mexican side of the border, there are good places to shop, whether you're looking for expensive items or a bargain.

To the north, along I-19, is the **Tubac Presidio Historical State Park,** site of the first military base in Arizona, established during the days of the Spanish exploration. Today there is a cathedral and a museum that houses artifacts from the Spanish colonial period.

At the **Tumacarori National Monument,** (602) 398-2341, on I-19, nineteen miles north of Nogales, are the remains of the abandoned mission of San Jose de Tumacarori. A museum nearby chronicles the story of the mission and of Spanish exploration.

Event: Mendocino Coast Whale Festival
When: Third (Mendocino) and fourth
(Fort Bragg) weekends in March
Where: Mendocino–Fort Bragg, California

Contact: Fort Bragg–Mendocino Coast Chamber of Commerce
P.O. Box 1141
Fort Bragg, CA 95437
(707) 964-3153

Something about the event: This event—actually two events held on successive weekends—takes place during the spring whale-watching season along the California coast. The first part, in Mendocino, features wine tastings and art exhibits. The second part, in Fort Bragg, includes a beer fest and wooden-boat show. Whale-watching excursions leave from both locales.

Accommodations with a personal touch:

Country Inn (I), 632 North Main Street, Fort Bragg, CA 95437, (707) 964-3737: 8 rms, pb, $60-95; cc-AE, MC, V; c-no, s-no, d-ltd, p-no, Cont Bkfst; h-Don and Helen Miller. House built in 1893 originally belonged to Union Lumber Company. Furnished with iron bedposts.

The Grey Whale Inn (I), 615 North Main Street, Fort Bragg, CA 95437, (707) 964-0640: 14 rms, pb, $60-125; c-ltd, s-ltd, d-yes, p-no, Full Bkfst (buffet); h-John and Colette Bailey. Redwood structure from 1915 features plants, comforters, and ocean view.

Joshua Grindle Inn (I), 44800 Little Lake Road, P.O. Box 647, Mendocino, CA 95460, (707) 937-4143: 10 rms, pb, $65-90; cc-AE, MC, V; c-over 10, s-no, d-no, p-no, Full Bkfst; h-Bill and Gwen Jacobson. House turned inn was built in 1879. It is furnished with antiques to match the period. State park nearby.

Mendocino Village Bed and Breakfast (I), Main Street, Box 626, Mendocino, CA 95460, (707) 937-0246: 12 rms, 10 pb, $55-110; cc-MC, V; c-ltd, s-ltd, d-no, p-no, Full Bkfst; h-Tom and Sue Allen. Wood-shingled inn from 1880s, formerly a doctor's office, now features antiques, seven fireplaces, and breakfast with homemade baked goods.

Roadside food: Quality seafood restaurants can be found in both Mendocino and Fort Bragg. The local seafood at **Cafe Beaujolais,** 961 Ukiah Street, (707) 937-5614, has been written up in gourmet magazines. **955,** at 955 Ukiah Street, (707) 937-1955, serves California cuisine. One highlight is baked red snapper in phyllo dough. At Fort Bragg, a seafood eatery of note is the **Wharf Restaurant,** 780 North Harbor Drive, (707) 964-4283

Some readings to enhance travels: Beck, Warren A., *California,* Doubleday, 1972; Federal Writers' Project, American Guide Series, *California: A Guide to the Golden Gate State,* 2d ed., Hastings, 1967; Hart, James D., *A Companion to California,* Oxford University Press, 1978; Lavender, David, *California,* Norton, 1976; Newcombe, Jack, *Northern California: A History and Guide: From Napa to Eureka,* Random House, 1986.

Berrill, Jacquelyn, *Wonders of Animal Migration,* Dodd, Mead, 1964; Burton, Robert, *The Life and Death of Whales,* Universe,

1973; McIntyre, Joan, *The Art of Whale Watching*, Sierra Club, 1982; Scheffer, Victor B., *The Year of the Whale*, Scribner, 1969.

Turn off here along the way: Mendocino's early settlers were from New England. The town's architecture is so plainly derived from New England's that Mendocino sometimes resembles a coastal town in Maine.

Mendocino is a community of artists. Local artwork is exhibited at the **Art Center,** 45200 Little Lake Road, (707) 937-5818.

In Fort Bragg, the **Stone Painting Museum** on S.R. 1, (707) 964-9450, displays works made from gems, petrified wood, and stone. Fort Bragg is also terminus for the "Skunk" railway of the **California Western Railroad.** Once a lumber line, it now carries excursion passengers in one car over a 40-mile journey to Wilkins. It's a train with personality.

Down the road at Little River, there is what's called a **pygmy forest.** Its pines and cypresses grow no higher than two feet because the soil is so highly acidic.

Mendocino and Fort Bragg are considered the gateway to the beautiful but rugged northern coast leading into Oregon. Some of the villages along the coast, such as **Ferndale** and **Eureka,** have Victorian architecture.

Event: Cherry Blossom and Japanese Culture Festival
When: First weekend in May
Where: Seattle, Washington

Contact: Cherry Blossom and Japanese Cultural Festival
Commission
P.O. Box 2476
Seattle, WA 98111
(206) 623-7900

Something about the event: This celebration of Japanese culture features traditional textiles, kimonos, art, games, and bonsai.

Accommodations with a personal touch:

The **Williams House** (B&B), 1505 Fourth Avenue North, Seattle, WA 98109, (206) 285-0810: 5 rms, pb, $45-60; cc-AE, DC, MC, V; c-yes, s-ltd, d-no, p-no, Full Bkfst; h-Susan and Doug Williams. Victorian home situated on Queen Anne Hill.

Galer Place (B&B), 318 West Galer Street, Seattle, WA 98105, (206) 282-5339: 4 rms, pb-2, $60-70; cc-AE, DC, MC, V; c-yes, s-ltd, d-no, p-yes, Full Bkfst. Victorian home from 1906 located near Seattle Center. Hot tubs on premises.

M.V. Challenger (B&B), 809 Fairview Place North, Seattle, WA 98109, (206) 340-1201: 4 cabins, pb-no, $60-75; cc-no; c-yes, s-no, d-no, p-no, Full Bkfst; h-Jerry Brown. Bunk-and-Breakfast on working tugboat moored at the south end of Lake Union. Stereo, oak interior, and fireplace.

Sorrento Hotel (H), 900 Madison Street, Seattle, WA 98104, (206) 622-6400: 76 rms, pb, $110-130; cc-AE, DC, DISC, MC, V; c-yes, s-yes, d-ltd, p-no, Cont Bkfst-ltd. Luxury hotel, built in 1908, offers traditional ambience with modern conveniences.

Pacific Bed and Breakfast (S), 701 Northwest 60th, Seattle, WA 98107, (206) 784-0539.

Roadside food: Salmon steaks, oysters, clams, and mussels are some of the items on the menus at Seattle seafood houses. They include **Fullers,** 1400 Sixth Avenue, (206) 621-9000; **Ray's Boat House,** 6049 Seaview Avenue Northwest, (206) 789-3770; and **F. X. McRory's Steak and Chop House,** 419 Occidental South, (206) 623-4800, where they age their beef for 32 days.

Some readings to enhance travels: Clark, Norman H., *Washington,* Norton, 1976; Faber, J. M., *An Irreverent Guide to Washington State,* Potter, 1981; Federal Writers' Project, American Guide Series, *Washington: A Guide to the Evergreen State,* Binford and Mort, 1941. For more books about Washington see "Fall Foliage Festival," page 210.

Araki, Nancy, and Horii, Jane, *Matsuri! Festival!: Japanese American Celebrations and Activities,* Heian Institute, 1985; Broom, Leonard, and Reimer, Ruth, *Removal and Return: The Socio-Economic Effects of War on Japanese-Americans,* University of California Press, 1974; Connor, John W., *Tradition and Change in Three Generations of Japanese Americans,* Nelson-Hall, 1977; Uchida, Yoshiko, *Desert Exile: The Uprooting of a Japanese-American Family,* University of Washington Press, 1982.

Turn off here along the way: The **Wing Luke Asian Museum,** 407 Seventh Avenue South, (206) 623-5124, documents the cultures of Asian communities in the Northwest. Exhibits include folk art, calligraphy, and photography.

Culture is prominent in Seattle. Throughout the year, the **Opera House** at **Seattle Center** is home to the **Seattle Opera** and to the **Northwest Ballet** and the **Seattle Symphony,** (206) 625-4234.

Also at the Seattle Center are the **Seattle Children's Museum,**

(206) 441-1767, a hands-on museum that encourages participants to touch and explore, and the tower known as the **Space Needle,** (206) 443-2100, which offers panoramic views of the lakes, the Cascade and Olympic Mountains, and, of course, Puget Sound.

It is the water that is Seattle's real pride and joy. **Pike Place Market,** Pike Street and First Avenue, (206) 682-7453, offers fish, vegetables, music, and old-time ambience. Nearby, along the piers, are the **Seattle Aquarium** on Pier 59, where you can observe shore animals in their underwater habitats, the **Omnidome Film Experience,** Pier 53, (206) 622-1868, a movie in the round; and **Pier 36,** (206) 286-5650, the departure point for ferries to the nearby islands and Canada.

Event: Jumpin' Frog Jubilee
When: Third weekend in May
Where: Angels Camp, California

Contact: 39th District Agricultural Association
P.O. Box 96
Angels Camp, CA 95222
(209) 736-2561

Something about the event: Mark Twain's short story "The Celebrated Jumping Frog of Calaveras County" inspired the annual frog-jumping contest at the Calaveras County Fair. Jumping frogs is a finely skilled art, and the contest draws competitors and spectators from far away. There is even a Rent-a-Frog booth.

Accommodations with a personal touch:

Dunbar House (I), 271 Jones Street, Box 1375, Murphys, CA 95247, (209) 728-2897: 5 rms, pb, $50-60; cc-no; c-yes, s-ltd, d-no, p-no, Cont Bkfst; h-John and Barbara Carr. Italianate inn with three-sided porch located on the main street. Antiques, lace, and fresh-cut flowers.

Murphys Hotel (H), 457 Main Street, P.O. Box 329, Murphys, CA 95247, (209) 728-3444: 29 rms, 22 pb, $48-68; cc-AE, MC, V; c-yes, s-yes, d-no, p-yes, Bkfst-no. Classic Old West hotel with saloon. President Grant stayed here soon after hotel opened in 1856.

Sutter Creek Inn (I), 75 Main Street, P.O. Box 385, Sutter Creek, CA 95685, (209) 267-5606: 19 rms, pb, $35-90; cc-no; c-no, s-ltd, d-no, p-no, Full Bkfst. Inn, built in 1859, features swinging beds, Franklin stoves, fireplaces, wicker, and old-style breakfast.

Roadside food: Hotel Lefers, 8404 Main Street, Maelumne Hill, (209) 286-1401, is an 1860s landmark hotel (the town, once a center of the gold rush, lost the election for state capital by a single vote). The menu is continental, with a French touch; the ribs are superior. Also in the area is the **Black Bart Inn,** 35 Main Street, San Andreas, (209) 754-3808, named after a famous stagecoach robber. It is now famous for its fish—so famous, in fact, that you can expect to wait in line on the weekends.

Some readings to enhance travels: Moore, Charles and Kristin, *The Mother Lode: Pictorial Guide to California's Gold Rush Country,* Chronicle, 1983; Yaeden, David, *Exploring Small Towns,* Ward Ritchie, 1973; Blasingame, Wyatt, *Wonders of Frogs and Toads,* Dodd, Mead, 1975; Cole, Joanna, *A Frog's Body,* William Morrow, 1980; Donaldson, Gerald, ed., *Frogs,* Van Nostrand Reinhold, 1980; Dickerson, Mary C.,*Frog Book,* Dover, 1969. See also "Mendocino Coast Whale Festival," page 185.

Turn off here along the way: Angels Camp is located in California's Mother Lode District, an area made prosperous by gold mining. The harsh world of the gold prospectors is reflected in the names of local towns, such as **Rough and Ready** and **Savage.** Although fewer and fewer old structures still survive, much of the area's history and flavor are preserved at **Big Oak Flat.** In season, you can catch a show of the period at the **Fallon Theater** in Columbia, 11185 Washington Street (Columbia State Park), (209) 946-2116.

In Mariposa, you can see the **Oldest Courthouse,** 5088 Bullion Street, (209) 966-3222. Dating back to 1854, it was built of white pine and constructed with wooden pegs. There are original furnishings and a bell tower transported from the east via Cape Horn.

Wineries dot the region. They include **Stevenot Wineries** in Murphys, 5690 San Domingo Road, (209) 728-3436; **Generic Wines,** 321 Spring Street, Nevada City, (916) 265-9463; and **Boeger Wineries** in Placerville, 1709 Carson Road, (916) 622-8094.

One of the area's greatest attractions is nature. **Big Tree State Park** sports the widest redwoods in the world—some reach 20 to 30 feet in diameter. One measured so wide that a dance floor was built on its stump. There are also caves and caverns. At **Moaning Cavern** near Ballcito, you can, if you're so inclined, rappel down for 180 feet. **Mercer Caves,** near Murphys, was found 100 years ago.

Event: Fleet of Flowers
When: Memorial Day
Where: Depoe Bay, Oregon

Contact: Memorial Day Fleet
P.O. Box 123
Depoe Bay, OR 97341
(503) 765-2345

Something about the event: Since 1945, crowds from throughout the country have gathered to witness the assembly of the flotilla on Memorial Day. Boats are decorated with flowers. A procession goes to the ocean, where wreaths are cast to commemorate loved ones lost at sea.

Accommodations with a personal touch:
   Ocean House (B&B), 4920 Northwest Woody Way, Newport, OR 97365, (602) 265-6158: 4 rms, 2 pb, $40-70; cc-MC, V; c-over 12, s-ltd, d-no, p-no, Full Bkfst; h-Bette and Bob Gerard. Home overlooking ocean features fireplace and deck.
   Channel House (I), P.O. Box 56, Depoe Bay, OR 97341, (503) 765-2140: 11 rms, pb, $40-140; cc-MC, V; c-yes, s-yes, d-yes, p-ltd, Full Bkfst; h-Paul Schwabe. B&B located at entrance to ocean. Ocean-view terraces and whirlpools.
   Northwest Bed and Breakfast (S), 7707 Southwest Locust Street, Portland, OR 97223, (602) 246-8366.

Roadside food: Depoe Bay is home to **Oceans Apart,** Highway 101, (503) 765-2513, which features cohos, salmon, halibut, and rock cod with "a touch of Hawaiian." The **Sea Hag,** Highway 101, (503) 765-2734, has offered superior seafood for 25 years and features Gracie Strom, a local lady who is something of a legend. She entertains diners using bottles as musical instruments. A unique experience.

Readings to enhance travels: Alt, David, and Hyndman, Donald, *Roadside Geology of Oregon,* Mountain Press, 1978; Donald, Marje, *Exploring the Oregon Coast by Car,* Image Imprints, 1978; Mainwaring, William L., *Exploring the Oregon Coast,* Westridge, 1985.
   Scott, Geoffrey, *Memorial Day* (for children), Carolrhoda, 1983; Ainsworth, Catherine H., *American Calendar Customs,* Clyde Press, 1980; Schaun, George and Virginia, *American Holidays and Special Days,* Maryland Historical Press, 1985.

Turn off here along the way: Depoe Bay is situated along the beautiful Oregon Coast on US 101.

The beach is famous for camping, hiking, clamming, crabbing, and scavenging. Moreover, the region is a fisherman's delight, with saltwater angling in the ocean and fishing in freshwater in the state parks just across the road.

Sea urchins, sea lions, and birds occupy **Otter Rock** and **Seal Rock.**

Just south of Yachats, **Cape Perpetuum** offers panoramic views of the ocean and coastline from 800 feet up.

SUMMER

Sand Castles in the Air

For many children, summer means days at the beach building sand castles. By September, when school starts, the pails, shovels, and surf are usually forgotten.

But some people never stop building in the sand. They are the ones who have transformed child's play into an art form.

Members of this group may be found at work on both coasts. Some are young, some old. Some mold sand as a diversion, others for their livelihood.

Imperial Beach near San Diego is known as the unofficial home of sand sculpturing. Each July (the exact date depends on the tide levels each year), Imperial Beach hosts the U.S. Open Sandcastle Competition (see page 195), bringing together sand sculptors in seven categories and offering over $15,000 in prizes.

What started as a small gathering in 1980 quickly grew into a major event in Southern California, drawing 150,000 competitors and spectators from as far away as British Columbia and land-locked Scottsdale, Arizona.

Although their tools are more elaborate than a plastic shovel and pail, many sand sculptors use implements that can be found in any kitchen or garage: spades, buckets, sticks, carving devices, measuring cups, and wine strainers. At the competition, the rules require that sculpting be done manually, without power tools. Masonry, garden, or household hand tools, a wheelbarrow, one ladder per team, pails, buckets, watering cans, and hand pump sprayers are all acceptable.

Moreover, sand sculptors must follow particular guidelines. For example, the structure must be formed within a designated 30-foot-square section, materials must be biodegradable (seaweed, shells), and no adhesives or glues may be used to hold the creation together.

An important consideration is always the location and type of sand. Some beaches, according to California architect and sand sculptor Kent Tollen, are better suited to sand sculpturing than others. "The higher the silt content," says Tollen, "the better the sand holds."

To Tollen, as well as to Gary Consella, an engineer, potter, and 3D artist from Escondido, California, questions of location and sand texture are of no small consequence. To them, it is more than just a matter of pride. A lot of dollars are on the line for these people. They are professional sand sculptors.

Consella and his team have created some of the most elaborate sand structures ever built, including Gothic cathedrals and Tudor castles. They created one "village" on a British Columbia beach that stood 50 feet high, covered an area the size of a football field, and required tour guides to lead visitors through. "The planning on blueprints alone can take up to a year," Consella says.

The novelty and artistry of intricate sand sculptures often bring business to a beach community. Executives frequently contract with sand sculptors to create messages in the sand. Some clients pay as much as half a million dollars.

Consella's professional sand sculpturing endeavors have taken him around the world. Officials in Japan flew him over to launch a sand sculpturing festival there. He has also constructed sand castles on the "Today Show." His clients have included a major auto manufacturer, for whom he built a full-size model in sand, and the San Diego Tourist Board, for whom he builds sand castles at travel industry conventions. "We stop them dead in their tracks," he says, "because we're so different."

In jobs done for corporations, technique is not as important as the final product. If local sand, for example, is not adequate, better sand will be shipped in. And because finished works may weigh thousands of pounds, shovels and pails just won't do. Instead, tractors and hydraulic jackhammers are brought in to get the job done. These techniques have spawned a debate between the pragmatists (those whose main goal is to get the job done) and the purists (for whom the means are as important as the end product).

Betsy and David Peterson compete at Imperial Beach, but their methods of sculpturing are quite different. They are amateurs who bring friends together to sculpt for the fun of it.

"We happened to be on the beach when the competition was taking place a few years ago," says Betsy. "As soon as we saw it, we said we had to participate."

Even though Betsy doubts their work can hold a candle to that of the professionals, she is careful to point out that their methods are not improvised either. Her husband, David, an architect, draws up blueprints. Stations are appointed, tools prepared. Technique is stressed, but to Betsy, the key is teamwork.

"We line up pails and tools, and make it clear that everyone's job, from bucket person up, is as crucial as the next," she says.

Both professional Gary Consella and amateur Betsy Peterson agree, however, that the secret to success in sculpturing is to use water properly.

"There are particular techniques in getting the sand to perform," Consella revealed. "You want to achieve the same compact consistency in air as when you walk on the beach, at water's edge."

Now where's that old sand shovel?

Event: U.S. Open Sandcastle Competition
When: Third weekend in July
Where: Imperial Beach, California

Contact: Sandcastle Days
825 Imperial Beach Boulevard
Imperial Beach, CA 92032
(619) 424-3151

Something about the event: Sand sculptors compete for the champion's title in both professional and amateur categories. In addition, there are fireworks, parades, and crafts.

Accommodations with a personal touch:
Britt House (I), 406 Maple Street, San Diego, CA 92103, (619) 234-2926: 9 rms, pb-no, $95-115; cc-AE, V; c-ltd, s-no, d-ltd, p-no, Full Bkfst; h-Don Martin. Victorian inn features stained glass, full breakfasts, and afternoon tea.

Harbor Hill Guest House (B&B), 2330 Albatross Street, San Diego, CA 92101, (619) 233-0638: 5 rms, pb, $50-70 ($10 each additional adult); cc-no; c-yes, s-yes; d-no, p-no, Cont Bkfst; h-Dorothy Milbourn. Old Spanish-style building near San Diego Zoo and Balboa Park. Ten minutes to Tijuana.

Heritage Park Bed and Breakfast (I), 2470 Heritage Park Row, San Diego, CA 92110, (619) 295-7088: 9 rms, pb, $75-115; cc-MC, V; c-over 12, s-no, d-yes, p-no, Full Bkfst; h-Lori Chandler. Inn, built in 1869, offers full breakfast, seacoast view, afternoon social hour (wine, cider, and appetizer), and old-time movies at night.

Carolyn's Bed and Breakfast Homes in San Diego (S), P.O. Box 84776, San Diego, CA 92138, (619) 435-5009.

Roadside food: San Diego touches two worlds, the ocean to the west and Mexico to the south. **Anthony's Harborside,** 1355 Harbor Road, (619) 232-6358, is a seafood restaurant specializing in sculpin, sea bass, abalone, halibut, fish and chips, and chowder. A taste of Mexico can be had at **El Indio Shop,** 3695 India Street, (619) 299-0333. It is a take-out restaurant—part of a factory that produces tortilla chips—that specializes in Sonoran-style Mexican food (less spicy than other kinds). Their tostadas are recommended.

Some readings to enhance travels: Lawson, Greg, *San Diego*, First Choice, 1986; Mills, James R., *San Diego, Where California Began*, San Diego Historical Society, 1985; Pryde, Phillip, *San Diego: An Introduction to the Region*, Kendall-Hunt, 1983.

Adkins, Jan, *Art and Industry of Sandcastles*, Water, 1982; Batho, Margot, *Sandcastling*, Lerner, 1973; Marks, Mickey Klar, *Sand Sculpturing*, Dial Press, 1962; Simo, Connie, et al., *Sanditiquity*, Taplinger, 1980.

Turn off here along the way: The beach and the sand-castling activities will likely keep you occupied for one full day. But there is much to visit elsewhere.

Along the water are the **U.S. Coast Guard Navy Training Center** and **Naval Air Station,** (619) 235-3534. Naval vessels can be toured at Saturday Open Houses. The **Maritime Museum of San Diego,** North Harbor Drive, (619) 234-9153, displays historic vessels and exhibits related to the sea.

The origins of San Diego are commemorated at the **Cabrillo National Monument** overlooking the harbor, (619) 557-5450. This is where the explorer Juan Rodriguez Cabrillo entered San Diego harbor for the first time in 1542. His arrival is reenacted every September. The streets of **Old Town,** (619) 237-6770, contain buildings from the mid-19th century. Today, San Diego has grown in every direction.

Culture plays a prominent role in San Diego today. **Balboa Park** is a recreational area that houses the **Botanical Gardens,** north of Lilac Pond, (619) 236-5717, the **Natural History Museum,** east end of El Prato, (619) 232-3821, the **Museum of Photographic Arts,** Casa de Balboa Building, (619) 239-5262, and the **San Diego Museum of Art,** center of park, (619) 232-7931.

Popular culture is on display at the **Lawrence Welk Museum** at nearby Escondido, (619) 749-2737, which traces the career of the man who made champagne music famous.

The world-famous **San Diego Zoo,** Zoo Drive, (619) 234-3153, contains 800 species totaling 3,200 animals, including some very rare species. The zoo has won critical acclaim for its thoughtful layout.

San Diego provides numerous recreational opportunities. Among them is the **Hotel del Coronado,** 1500 Orange Avenue, Coronado, (619) 435-6611, a century-old beach resort, famous for its Victorian architecture and rumored to be the first meeting place of the Duke of Windsor and Wallis Simpson.

A light rapid transit system (trolley) runs between downtown San Diego and Tijuana, Mexico. It is only a short ride, but the two cities are worlds apart.

Event: Gilroy Garlic Festival
When: Third weekend in July
Where: Gilroy, California

Contact: Gilroy Garlic Festival
P.O. Box 2311
Gilroy, CA 95201
(408) 842-1625

Something about the event: The "Garlic Capital of the World" draws an international spectrum of cooks and garlic lovers. In addition to garlic-cooking competitions, there is a 200-booth gourmet alley, plus garlic braids, wreaths, jewelry, T-shirts, and cookbooks.

Accommodations with a personal touch:

Mangels House (B&B), P.O. Box 302, Aptos, CA 95001, (408) 688-7982: 5 rms, pb-no, $84-98; cc-MC, V; c-over 12, s-ltd, d-no, p-ltd, Full Bkfst; h-Jamie Fisher. Inn, built in 1886, on the coast with a mountain view.

Bayview Hotel (H), 8041 Soquel Drive, Aptos, CA 95003, (408) 688-8654: 16 rms, 6 pb, $55; cc-MC, V; c-yes, s-yes, d-no, p-no, Cont Bkfst. Oldest hotel in the area, near the beach.

Babbling Brook Inn (I), 1025 Laorec Street, Santa Cruz, CA 95060, (408) 427-2437: 12 rms, pb, $85-125; cc-AE, DISC, MC, V; c-over 12, s-ltd, d-yes, p-no, Full Bkfst; h-Tom and Helen King. Inn from 1909. Gardens in European style.

Darling House (I), 314 West Cliff Drive, Santa Cruz, CA 95056, (408) 458-1958: 8 rms, 2 pb, $65-160; cc-MC, V; c-ltd, s-ltd, d-ltd, p-no, Cont Bkfst; h-Karen Darling. Oceanside mansion from 1910, with glass, antiques, and fireplaces. All rooms have ocean views.

Roadside food: The **Salmon Poacher,** 3035 Main Street, Soquel, (408) 476-1556, features salmon, trout, clams, oysters, mussels, and scallops. At the **Sea Cloud,** Municipal Wharf, Santa Cruz, (408) 458-9393, the menu changes daily, but you can always find mesquite-grilled fish with nouvelle-cuisine sauces.

Some readings to enhance travels: Braida, Charlene A., *Glorious Garlic: A Cookbook,* Stoney Communications, 1986; Doeser, Linda, and Richardson, Rosamond, *The Little Garlic Book,* Harris, 1983. See also "Mendocino Coast Whale Festival," page 184.

Turn off here along the way: The area around Gilroy is dotted with wineries. One is the **Pedrizzetti Winery,** located at 1645 San Pedro Avenue in Morgan Hill, (408) 779-7389.

The Spanish colonial influence in California can be seen at the **San Juan Bautista Mission,** Second and Meriposa Streets, (408) 623-4528, built in 1797. Indian carvings may be seen in the mission's interior.

To the north, San Jose and the Santa Clara Valley have long histories. Today the area has come to be known as **Silicon Valley** for the many high-tech, silicon-based companies that have made it their home.

Railway enthusiasts can ride between Felton and Santa Cruz the way it used to be done during the golden age of railroading on the **Santa Cruz Big Trees and Pacific Railroad,** (408) 335-4484. There is also a narrow-gauge railway that carries passengers among the redwoods.

At approximately the same time of year as the Garlic Festival in Gilroy, neighbors to the north in Santa Cruz put on a Calamari Festival (August). Add a little wine and Italian bread and you've got a real feast. For information, call (408) 423-6927.

Event: Loggers' Jubilee
When: Second weekend in August
Where: Morton, Washington

Contact: Loggers' Jubilee
P.O. Box 436
Morton, WA 98356
(206) 498-5250

Something about the event: Morton has been a logging community since 1891. The Loggers' Jubilee offers competitions in more than 15 events, including speed climbing and tree topping.

Accommodations with a personal touch:
   National Park Inn (I), Route 706, Longmire, WA (mail: Mount Rainier Guest Services Inc., Star Route, Ashford, WA 98304), (206) 569-2275: 16 rms, 9 pb, $35-49; cc-MC, V; c-yes, s-yes, d-no, p-no, Bkfst-no (available in restaurant). Inn is a 1920 rustic log building, situated in the midst of Mount Rainier National Park near hiking trails. An extended drive from Morton.

Roadside food: The area used to be famous for its lumberjack breakfast eateries, but today the only place where such a breakfast can be found is at the festival itself, on one morning. Check at the event for details. The **Wheel Cafe–Jubilee Room,** Main Street, (206) 496-3240, serves wholesome food, and features steak.

Some readings to enhance travels: Corrigan, George, *Caulked Boots and Cart Hooks,* Coronet, 1986; Smith, Robert, *My Life in the North Woods,* Atlantic Monthly, 1986; Sorden, L. G., and Vallier, Jacques, *Lumber Jack Lingo,* Northwood, 1986; Williams, Richard L., *The Loggers,* Time-Life, 1976. See also "Cherry Blossom and Japanese Culture Festival," page 187.

Turn off here along the way: On Hopkins Hill, to the west of Morton, you can catch a view of the **Mount St. Helens Crater.** The area around the crater has been designated a National Volcanic Monument. It covers 110,000 acres destroyed by the 1980 volcano. Access to the area is limited. Among the accessible locations are North America's largest lava tube (a 12,000-foot tunnel) and the Visitors' Center, 3029 Spirit Lake Highway, Castle Rock, (206) 274-6644, which shows films and model volcano displays.
   The headquarters of **Mount Rainier National Park** are located on the Star Route, Ashford, WA 98304, (206) 569-2211. The 14,000-

foot peak is the highest in the Northwest. There are 140 miles of roads and 300 miles of forest trails open to the public. But don't get too comfortable. Mount Rainier is a volcano, which, they say, could blow like Mount St. Helens at any time.

Event: Bat Flight Breakfast
When: Mid-August
Where: Carlsbad, New Mexico

Contact: Carlsbad Caverns National Park
3225 National Parks Highway
Carlsbad, NM 88220
(505) 785-2232

Something about the event: An alfresco predawn breakfast at the mouth of the caves precedes the yearly return of the 500,000 freetail bats who roost there.

Accommodations with a personal touch:
   The Lodge (I), U.S. 82, Box 497, Cloudcroft, NM 88317, (505) 682-2566: 58 rms, pb, $49-150; cc-AE, MC, V; c-yes, s-yes, d-ltd, p-no, Cont Bkfst; h-Judy Montoly. Lodge, situated on scenic summit, was first built by a railroad. Resort-type accommodations. An extended drive from Carlsbad.

Roadside food: You can have a taste of barbecue and the Old West at the **Flying Chuck Wagon**, 7505 Old Canyon Highway, (505) 887-9996. There is entertainment too. If you can do without the entertainment, **Full House Restaurant**, 810 Canal Street, (505) 887-2724, serves recommended prime ribs.

Some readings to enhance travels: Looney, Ralph, *Haunted Highways*, University of New Mexico Press, 1979; Federal Writers' Project, American Guide Series, *New Mexico: A Guide to the Colorful State*, rev. ed., Hastings, 1962; Sinclair, Marc, *New Mexico*, Norton, 1977.
   Barbour, Roger W., and Davis, Wayne H., *Bats of America*, University Press of Kentucky, 1979 (reprint of 1969 ed.); Yalden, D. W., and Morris, P. A., *The Lives of Bats*, Times, 1976; Mohr, Charles E., *The World of the Bat*, J. B. Lippincott, 1926; Peterson, Russell, *Silently by Night*, McGraw-Hill, 1964.

Turn off here along the way: The caverns in **Carlsbad National Park** were formed millions of years ago by the percolation of groundwater into limestone. Unique plant life and rock formations appear in a variety of forms. Self-guided tours are available. Information can be acquired at the Visitors Center, (505) 785-2232. Samples of the minerals and plant life can be seen in town at the library of the **Carlsbad Museum,** 101 South Halvaguero, (505) 885-6776.

At the **Antique Auto Barn,** National Parks Highway, (505) 885-2457, 40 antique cars have been restored and placed on display.

To the north is **Artesia,** a town known for underground resources. Its water was pumped for irrigation, artesian wells and its oil was pumped for fuel. It even sports an underground school built to withstand a nuclear war (White Sands Ranch Missile Site is not far away.)

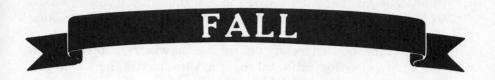

FALL

Fruit of the Vine

Its production is based on techniques that go back to antiquity. It has been an inspiration for artists and a potion for lovers. Wine holds a special place in people's hearts.

Over the past 15 years, there has been a renaissance in wine consumption and consequently in wine production. Today, liquor stores carry wine not only from France and Italy, the traditional sources of wine, but from Portugal and other Mediterranean countries, as well as from American wineries. Domestically, there has been a boom in wineries both large and small. They have developed to fulfil the growing demand for table wines and for the newer products such as wine coolers.

The larger commercial wineries, such as Ernest and Julio Gallo and Taylor Wines, cater to national mass markets. Their techniques are very different from those used by traditional French wine makers in the Loire Valley. "Those big wineries make wine like an oil company would produce their product at a refinery," muses one small-scale wine maker. At many vineyards across the country, including several in California's Napa Valley and New York's Finger Lakes region, there are wine makers who practice their trade the old-fashioned way, storing wine in wood barrels.

On the whole, however, a combination of old-time values and modern methods prevails. "Anyone not using technology today would be crazy," says Louis Fappiano, a fourth-generation member of a family that has operated the Fappiano Winery in California since 1896. "Winemaking continues to be an ongoing evolution, as it has been over three thousand years. There is no such thing as old-fashioned in today's world."

Fappiano explains that he and other area wineries rely heavily on the expertise of chemists at the University of California at Davis in producing their cabernet sauvignon and zinfandel. If modern aids were ignored and bacteria were to sneak through, says Fappiano, "I could be left with 50 percent vinegar instead of wine."

Despite the modern techniques used at his winery, Fappiano says that the family vineyards still maintain tradition. "There's no set recipe to making good wine," he says. "The process is still subjective and it is the wine maker, not a formula, that determines whether a wine will be a success."

At the Frey Winery in California's Midwood Valley, the wine-making techniques are unusual not so much for being old-fashioned as for being organic. "We don't use any herbicides, pesticides, or other chemicals in the grape-growing process," explains Paul Frey.

Frey did not enter the business with the kind of driving ambition that motivates many growers. He had built a second home in Mendocino and started growing grapes there in 1967 for the tax benefits.

It was his eight sons (he is the father of twelve) who turned an avocation into a commercial endeavor by applying the expertise they had acquired at other wineries.

"I was indifferent, but they have made it happen with some old dairy equipment, lots of hard work, and without a lot of working capital," Frey says.

Today, the winery is doing well at a production level of six thousand bottles each year, says Frey. That's nowhere near the eight hundred thousand produced annually at a nearby winery, but there are other rewards. Pope John Paul II drank Frey wine when he visited California. Apparently, the Archbishop of San Francisco's cook selected it after he tasted a sample at a wine shop and liked it.

A crowd of wine lovers indulges in an old-fashioned grape stomp each September at the Delicato Vineyards at Manteca, California (see "Delicato Grape Stomp," page 205). On the Sunday of Labor Day weekend, folks come by the thousands to press grapes with their feet, the way it was done before the age of machinery. The stompers are aided by the strains of traditional Italian accordion music. There are also arts and crafts, food and wine booths, antique cars, and other amusement.

Health regulations prohibit the stomped grapes from being turned into wine, but for most participants the stomp is an occasion to try something unique. The process is tougher than it looks. "There is more to it than just jumping on grapes," says Dorothy Indelicato of the Vineyards. "There's a drain there, so stomping is only part of the process—the other part is getting the juice out."

Even here, tradition has had to be modified. Instead of using their bare feet, the stompers wear tennis shoes for their own protection. Each year a champion is crowned. But ribbons and trophies do not impress everyone, says Indelicato.

"Some of the old-timers who actually stomped on grapes in the old country are up there in years," she says, "so they don't crush anymore. But they make it clear what they feel the correct technique is."

It's a technique that worked for several thousand years.

Event: Delicato Grape Stomp
When: First weekend in September
Where: Manteca, California

Contact: Delicato Grape Stomp
12001 South Highway 99
Manteca, CA 95336
(209) 239-1215

Something about the event: In addition to an old-fashioned grape stomp, this harvest celebration offers food booths, entertainment, arts and crafts, antique cars, and tours of the winery.

Accommodations with a personal touch:
   Ambert House (B&B), 1315 22d Street, Sacramento, CA 95816, (916) 444-8085: 4 rms, 2 pb, $70-95; cc-AE, MC, V; c-no, s-no, p-no, d-no, Full Bkfst; h-Jane and Michael Richardson. Sitting room, library, stained glass, and gourmet breakfasts.
   Aunt Abigail's Bed and Breakfast (B&B), 2120 G Street, Sacramento, CA 95816, (916) 441-5007: 5 rms, pb, $55-80; cc-AE, DC, MC, V; c-ltd, s-no, d-no, p-no, Full Bkfst; h-Susanne Ventura. Turn-of-the-century mansion near State Capitol. Fresh flowers and mints.
   Bear Flag Inn (B&B), 2814 I Street, Sacramento, CA 95816, (916) 448-5714: 4 rms, 2 pb, $59-83; cc-AE, DC, MC, V; c-over 5, s-no, d-no, p-no, Full Bkfst; h-Dean Wofford. Restored 1915 home near downtown. Antiques, books, and fireplaces.
   Briggs House (B&B), 2209 Capitol, Sacramento, CA 95816, (916) 441-3214: 7 rms, 4 pb, $60-95; cc-AE, MC, V; c-ltd, s-no, d-ltd, p-no, Full Bkfst. Colonial-style B&B. Gourmet breakfasts, jacuzzi, and sauna.

Roadside food: There are a number of good Sacramento eateries. At **Lautrec's**, 545 Monroe Street, (916) 973-0403, the menu is

French, highlighted by New Zealand venison. **Sal's,** 2008 Sutterville Road, (916) 454-9404, serves Mexican food that is described as "down and dirty." They are famous for their fajitas as well as for a salsa bar whose food ranges from mild to hot. For nouvelle cuisine, there are **Scooner's,** 28th and N Streets, (916) 452-7427, and **Pava,** 24th and K Streets, (916) 443-2397, where the portions are unusually hefty. In Old Sacramento is the **Cafe La Salle,** 1028 Second Street, (916) 442-9000, which specializes in Beef Wellington and onion soup.

Some readings to enhance travels: Bachelis, Faren Marie, *Pelican Guide to Sacramento, The Gold Country,* Pelican, 1987; Kaufman, William I., *The Traveler's Guide to the Vineyards of North America,* Penguin, 1980; Wagner, Phillip M., *Grapes into Wine: The Art of Winemaking in America,* Knopf, 1976; Wagenvourd, James, *The Wine Book,* Putnam, 1976; Weaver, Robert J., *Grape Growing,* Wiley, 1976. See also "Mendocino Coast Whale Festival," page 185.

Turn off here along the way: Although it is less well known than some other wine-making parts of the state, Manteca, located in the San Joaquin Valley not far from the Pacific Coast and I-5, has been at it for 120 years.

Wineries dot the countryside. **Lodi** hosts a Grape Festival and Wine Show each September.

Stockton is a regional center and a deep-channel port. The history of the region is displayed at the **Haggin Museum,** 1201 Pershing Avenue, (209) 462-4116.

To the south is **Modesto,** the place that inspired the movie *American Graffiti.* Each year, the movie and Modesto are celebrated on American Graffiti night (second weekend in June).

To the east is **Yosemite National Park,** whose beauty draws naturalists and tourists alike. Also to the east are the California Hills, gold country.

Event: Albuquerque International Balloon Fiesta
When: First few weekends in October
Where: Albuquerque, New Mexico

Contact: Albuquerque International Balloon Fiesta
4804 Hawkins Northeast
Albuquerque, NM 87109
(505) 344-3501

Something about the event: Cutter Balloonpart, named after the event's founder, Sid Cutter, is a scene of wonder as hundreds of beautiful balloons fill the skies over Albuquerque. Tens of thousands come to watch. The event has helped make the region a mecca for balloonists from around the world.

Accommodations with a personal touch:
  Casita Chamisa (B&B), 850 Chamisa Road Northwest, Albuquerque, NM 87107, (505) 897-4644: 2 rms, pb, $50-95; cc-MC, V; c-yes, s-ltd, d-ltd, p-ltd, Cont Bkfst; h-Arnold and Kit Sargent. Historic adobe house on archeological site near Old Town. One host is an archeologist who provides tours.
  Apple Tree Inn (B&B), P.O. Box 787, Cedar Crest, NM 87008, (505) 281-3092: 2 rms, 1 pb, $45-90; cc-no; c-yes, s-yes, d-yes, p-ltd, Cont-Plus Bkfst; h-Norma Greimer. Deluxe accommodations in traditional adobe casita. Secluded, off the beaten path, but near Albuquerque.

Roadside food: Albuquerque's culinary scene is generally dominated by Mexican flavors. At **Rancho de Corrales,** three miles north of Alameda Road, (505) 897-3131, the specialties arc Spanish as well as northern Mexican. **La Placita Dining Room,** 204 San Felipe Northwest, Albuquerque, (505) 247-2204, serves New Mexican food (predominantly with chiles) and American entrees. **Garduno's of Mexico,** 10551 Montgomery Northeast, (505) 298-5000, brings a bit of Mexico to New Mexico with such items as burritos and fajitas.

Some readings to enhance travels: Simmons, Marc, *Albuquerque: A Narrative History,* University of New Mexico Press, 1979.
  Crouch, Tom D., *The Eagle Aloft: Two Centuries of Ballooning in America,* Smithsonian, 1983; Norwood, Amogene B., *Taming the Gentle Giant: A Guide to Hot Air Ballooning,* Land O'Sky Aeronautics, 1986; Jackson, Donald D., et al., *The Aeronauts,* Time-Life, 1980; Wirth, Dick, and Young, Jerry, *Ballooning: The Complete*

Guide to Riding the Winds, Random House, 1980. See also "Bat Flight Breakfast," page 200.

Turn off here along the way: Spanish, Indian, and contemporary cultures converge in Albuquerque. Several sites in the area reflect this balance between old and new. Its **Old Town,** restored after years of neglect, dates back to 1706 and provides a sense of continuity in the face of the changes wrought by the growth of the local aerospace and defense industries. The old and the new are bonded by the awesome beauty of the surrounding mountains.

The **Albuquerque Museum,** 2000 Mountain Road, (505) 243-7255, chronicles the history of the Rio Grande Valley. The museum building itself is an early solar-heated structure.

Not far to the north lies Los Alamos, where the nuclear bomb was developed. The impact of nuclear weaponry can be seen at an exhibit at the **National Atomic Museum,** Kirkland Air Force Base, Albuquerque, (505) 844-8443.

Albuquerque is home to the **University of New Mexico.** The 7,000-acre campus includes the **Art Museum,** (505) 277-4001, and the **Museum of Anthropology,** (505) 277-4044.

To the east is **Sandia Peak,** a winter ski area. Year-round, its tram offers a panoramic view for miles around. You feel as if you were up in a balloon.

Event: Salmon Days
When: First weekend in October
Where: Issaquah, Washington

Contact: Chamber of Commerce
160 Northwest Gilman Boulevard
Issaquah, WA 98027
(206) 392-7024

Something about the event: Each year, the salmon return to Issaquah Creek to spawn. The festival celebrating their arrival features tours of salmon hatcheries, a parade, arts and crafts, music, dance, and sports.

Accommodations with a personal touch:
Colonial Inn (I), Fall City, WA 98024, (206) 222-5191: 6 rms, 1 pb, $25-32; cc-MC, V; c-ltd, s-yes, d-no, p-no, Bkfst-ltd; h-Ed and Helen DeGrave. A 1900s stopover along river, now a restaurant and inn.

The **Wildflower** (B&B), 25237 Southeast Issaquah–Fall City Road, Issaquah, WA 98027, (206) 747-6277: 4 rms, 3 pb, $35-45; cc-no; c-over 12, s-no, d-no, p-no, Full Bkfst. Authentic log cabin with gazebo, set in 12 acres of evergreens and walking paths. Antiques and quilts.

Roadside food: Harry O's, 719 Northwest Gilman Boulevard, Issaquah, (206) 392-8614, serves American cuisine, including steak and lobster. Special pride goes into the preparation of the Pacific salmon, especially during Salmon Days.

Some readings to enhance travels: Berrill, Jacquelyn, *Wonders of Animal Migration*, Dodd, Mead, 1964; Childerhose, R. J., and Trim, Margeret, *Pacific Salmon and Steelhead Trout*, University of Washington Press, 1979; Dennor, Jerry, *The Salmon Cookbook*, Pacific Search, 1978; Hogan, Paula Z., *The Salmon*, Raintree, 1979. See also "Cherry Blossom and Japanese Culture Festival," page 187.

Turn off here along the way: The village now known as Issaquah was created as a railroad town in the gold-mining boom. It was then called Gilman, but the name was changed before the turn of the century. You'll still find the Gilman name at a series of restored pioneer houses that are now restaurants and boutiques.

You can ride the rails as they used to be on the **Puget Sound and Snoqualmie Valley Railroad,** S.R. 202, (206) 746-4025. Steam engines and street cars run as a traveling museum on a seven-mile line.

Event: Fall Foliage Festival
When: Last weekend in September through first weekend in October
Where: Leavenworth, Washington

Contact: Chamber of Commerce
P.O. Box 327
Leavenworth, WA 98826
(509) 548-7914

Something about the event: Leavenworth looks like a village in Bavaria. It celebrates the season with German music, a parade, theater, art, sports, and, of course, German food and beer.

Accommodations with a personal touch:

Haus Rohrbach Pension (I), 12882 Ranger Road, Leavenworth, WA 98826, (509) 548-7024: 10 rms, pb-6, $50-80; cc-MC, V; c-yes, s-no, d-ltd, p-no, Full Bkfst; h-Bob Harrild. European-style country inn modeled after an Austrian inn.

Brown's Farm (F), 11150 Highway 209, Leavenworth, WA 98826, (509) 548-7863: 3 rms, pb-no, $45-65; cc-MC, V; c-yes, s-ltd, d-no, p-no, Full Bkfst; h-Wendi Krieg. Country farmhouse from 1910, with stained glass. Behind it is a national forest.

Traveler's Bed and Breakfast (S), P.O. Box 492, Mercer Island, WA 98040, (206) 232-2345.

Roadside food: Of the several German restaurants in town, two come especially recommended: **Edelweiss Restaurant,** 843 Front Street, (509) 548-7015, and **Rhiner's Gasthaus,** 829 Front Street, (509) 548-5111.

Some readings to enhance travels: *Leaves: One Hundred Seventy-Seven Photographs,* Dover, 1984; Prance, Ghillean T., *Leaves: The Formation, Characteristics, and Uses of Hundreds of Leaves Found in All Parts of the World,* Crown, 1985. For more on Washington see "Cherry Blossom and Japanese Culture Festival," page 187.

Fielder, John, *Washington, Magnificent Wilderness,* Westcliffe, 1986; O'Hara, Pat, *Washington Images of the Landscape,* Westcliffe, 1987; Thollander, Earl, *Back Roads of Washington,* Crown, 1981.

Turn off here along the way: The area surrounding Leavenworth is Lumber Country. Up the road from Leavenworth is **Gold Bar,** the site of anti-Chinese riots in mid-1800s.

The region is also famous for its fruits and nuts. The **Liberty Orchards,** 117 Mission Street, Leavenworth, (509) 782-2191, produces and mails fruit and nut products nationwide. Tours of the orchards and packing facilities are available.

WINTER

The Civilized Side to the Wild West

When a group of cowboys and cowgirls first assembled in Elko, Nevada, in 1985, they called the gathering a reunion, even though many of them had never met. They were entitled to some poetic license, however, because these cowpunchers were also poets.

The very notion of cowpuncher poetry seems contradictory to some people. The popular image of the cowherd is a rough-and-ready type who relies on brawn and doesn't have much use for literature. But there's more. There's a longstanding tradition of poetry on the range. The first known collection of cowherd poems was published in the 1890s.

According to James Griffith, director of the Southwest Folklore Center of the University of Arizona, "cowboy poetry" has been around at least as far back as the 1870s. "After all, cowboy children had to go to school, where they learned to memorize and recite poems," he says. In addition, cowhands are notoriously fond of singing. "What is a song," asks Griffith, "if not a poem that has been set to music? And what do you do if you like the story and the words, but can't carry a tune in a saddlebag? Some sing anyway, but others recite." Much of the poetry written on the range was set down in secret and was often kept hidden. It was not until a meeting of national folk artists took place in Washington, D.C., in the early 1980s that the idea of a gathering solely for cowhand poetry surfaced. After some discussion and exploration, the first Cowboy Poetry Gathering was held in 1985 (see page 213).

The gatherings draw two thousand cowboys, ranchers, and western enthusiasts—a diverse group with a common bond. They come from as far away as the Dakotas and Oregon, and range in age from 20 to 80. For many, it has been a revelation to discover that they are not alone. Hal Canyon, director of the Western Folklife

Center in Salt Lake City, says that one cowboy poet told him that he wrote poetry for years without realizing that anyone else did too.

One participant is Nyle Henderson of Hotchkiss, Colorado. He creates his poetry while breaking in horses on his family ranch. According to Henderson, it is something that comes naturally to him. "I never really thought much about my poetry till after I'd been writing it six or seven years," he explains. "It just seemed a satisfying way to communicate what I saw and felt."

The poetry read at the gathering reflects western life in all its aspects. There are romantic images of the wilderness in all its beauty, meditations on the isolation and harshness of the work.

Georgie Stickling, a poet from Nevada, speaks often of solitude in her poetry. "I guess it was loneliness that started me making up poems—living by myself, without much to read, I had a lot of time to think."

Stickling learned to ride at the age of two and was working as a farm hand at 16. After years of roping, mending fences, packing salt, and shoeing, Stickling now owns her own ranch, where she raises cows and writes poetry.

In addition to poetry, the gathering highlights western range culture generally, with western movies, folk crafts, music, and art.

Cowhand art occupies center stage at the Russell Museum in Great Falls, Montana, which possesses one of the largest collections of western American art. It is named for C. M. Russell, the first artist of note to paint the range from the perspective of the cowhands rather than from the perspective of eastern journalists and cartoonists.

Each March, the museum hosts an auction of art of the range, past and present (see "Western Art Auction," page 171). It is a popular event with artists, collectors, and those who feel that art is an especially powerful way of communicating what the West is about.

"These genre pictures restate some very basic things about life around cattle and the West," says Mike Korn of the Russell Museum. "The two traditions seem to grow out of one another like good braided rawhide."

Ron Hayes puts it another way. He is a self-taught cowboy artist. While he understands issues of tone, color, and other artistic questions, he describes the role of his art simply. "I paint because I like to, and I do cowboys because it's what I know best."

Event: Cowboy Poetry Gathering
When: Last weekend in January
Where: Elko, Nevada

Contact: Cowboy Poetry Gathering
P.O. Box 888
Elko, NV 89801
(701) 738-7508

Something about the event: Cowboys and cowgirls get together to read their poetry. In addition, there are western films, crafts, and art and music of the range.

Accommodations with a personal touch:
  Breitenstein House (B&B), General Delivery, Lamoille, NV 89828, (702) 753-6356: 4 rms, pb, $40-65; cc-MC, V; c-yes, s-yes, d-ltd, p-yes, Full Bkfst; h-Harold Ulrich. B&B with country atmosphere, set on 640-acre ranch against the mountains.
  Old Pioneer Garden (B&B), Star Route 79, Unionville, NV 89418, (702) 538-7585: 11 rms, 3 pb, $35-45; cc-no; c-yes, s-ltd, d-ltd, p-ltd, Full Bkfst; h-Mitzi and Len Jones. Old country inn with 1920–1930s vintage furniture, set on 120 acres. Extended drive to Elko.

Roadside food: The region is a center of Basque immigrant culture. The Basques were sheepherders in their homeland, the Pyrenees Mountains of France and Spain. Many have taken up the same occupation here. They have fiercely safeguarded their customs—and that includes food. **Golden Canal,** 1830 Idaho Street, Elko, (702) 738-3418, specializes in filet mignon; its dishes have a distinctively Spanish flavor. **Nevada,** 351 Silver Street, Elko, (702) 738-8485, features beef, including various cuts of steak (T-bone, top rib, and New York cut). **Star Restaurant,** 246 Silver Street, Elko, (702) 738-9925, is also recommended for its steak.

Some readings to enhance travels: Laxalt, Robert, *Nevada,* Norton, 1977; Toll, David W., *The Compleat Nevada Traveler,* University of Nevada Press, 1976.
  Dana, Bill, *Cowboy–English, English–Cowboy Dictionary,* Ballantine, 1982; Hoig, Stan, *The Humor of the American Cowboy,* University of Nebraska Press, 1970; Potter, Edgar F., *Cowboy Slang,* Golden West, 1986.

Turn off here along the way: Cowhands may be seen riding the roads near Elko. The town is in eastern Nevada, on I-80, in country variously known for its pioneers, ranchers, and miners. Mining can still be seen at **Copper Canyon** along I-80 as you drive westward toward Reno.

Elko is home to the National Basque Festival, which takes place every July. It is an occasion to celebrate Basque culture through music, consumption of lamb and other traditional Basque dishes, and games of strength. (See also "Basque Sheepherders' Ball and Lamb Auction," page 174.)

Event: Hopi Social Dances
When: January (dates vary)
Where: Hopi Reservation, Arizona

Contact: Hopi Cultural Center
P.O. Box 69
Second Mesa, AZ 86043
(602) 734-2401

Something about the event: The Hopi sponsor a variety of events that are open to the general public. In January, visitors are invited to attend the Buffalo Dance and other traditional dances. Traditional food is served in Hopi homes.

Accommodations with a personal touch:
   Walking L Ranch (B&B), R.R. 4, Box 721B, Flagstaff, AZ 86001, (602) 779-2219: 2 rms, pb-no, $30-40; cc-no; c-yes, s-ltd, d-no, p-no, Full Bkfst; h-Susan and Jerry Ladhoff. Ranch situated in national forest features hot tub, art studio, and horses.
   Dierker House (B&B), Flagstaff, AZ 86001, (602) 774-3249: 3 rms, pb-no, $26-40; cc-no; c-over 12, s-no, d-no, p-no, Full Bkfst; h-Dorothy Dierker. Guest kitchen and wine in refrigerator are some of the extra comforts at this B&B.

Roadside food: You can get a taste of Hopi culture at the **Hopi Cultural Center Restaurant,** Route 264, Second Mesa, (602) 734-2401. *Piki* bread, *nok qui vi* (stew of lamb, corn, chili, and fried bread), and cornmeal pancakes are but a few of the items on the menu. For the less adventurous, nontraditional entries such as French fries and sandwiches are on the menu too.

Some readings to enhance travels: Clemmer, Richard O., *Continuities of Hopi Culture Change*, Acoma, 1978; Courlander, Harold, ed., *Hopi Voices: Recollections, Traditions and Narratives of Hopi*

Indians, University of New Mexico Press, 1982; Harlow, Francis, *Introduction to Hopi Pottery*, Museum of Northern Arizona, 1978; Qoyawayma, Polingaysi, *No Turning Back: A Hopi Indian Woman's Struggle To Live in Two Worlds*, University of New Mexico Press, 1977. See also "Cinco de Mayo," page 184.

Turn off here along the way: Second Mesa is located in the lands set aside for the Hopi Nation in northeast Arizona. It's north of Winslow and east of the Grand Canyon. A visit should not be made without preparation. Roads can be slow and their condition variable. Before setting out, have your car checked, for there are few services in the area.

It is important to note that permission must be obtained in order to take photographs on reservation land, and there is a charge.

S.R. 264 is the main east–west thoroughfare through the Hopi Nation. It runs parallel and to the north of I-40. Along the way, it passes through villages and farms. You can learn about the area, its people, and specifically about the tribal culture at the **Hopi Cultural Center** east of Kykotsmovi, (602) 734-2401. There are displays and exhibits on Hopi history and crafts, including silverwork.

Among the Hopi villages are **Old Oraibi,** which has been occupied since the year 1100.

Event: San Ildefonso Pueblo Feast Day
When: Third week in January
Where: Pueblo Tribal Lands,
New Mexico (near Santa Fe)

Contact: San Ildefonso Pueblo
Route 5, Box 315A
Santa Fe, NM 87501
(505) 455-2273

Something about the event: Buffalo and deer dances are performed by the Pueblo Indians on this feast day. The pueblo is located 25 miles northwest of Santa Fe. The pottery on display is a tribal specialty.

Accommodations with a personal touch:
  La Posada de Chimayo (I), P.O. Box 463, Chimayo, NM 87522, (505) 351-4605: 2 rms, pb, $65 ($25 each additional person); cc-no; c-yes, s-yes, d-no, p-ltd, Full Bkfst; h-Sue Farrington. Traditional

adobe guest house located on high road between Santa Fe and Taos.

Orange Street Bed and Breakfast (I), 3496 Orange Street, Los Alamos, NM 87544, (505) 662-2651: 3 rms, pb-no, $25; cc-no; c-yes, s-no, d-no, p-no, Full Bkfst; h-Hester Sargent. House in town, filled with antiques.

Roadside food: Eateries using chile peppers in various forms can be found throughout the state. In Taos, **Casa de Valdez,** South Santa Fe Road, Taos, (505) 753-8777, features New Mexican cuisine, highlighted by steaks barbecued over a hickory pit. Mexican food is on the menu at the **Chile Connection,** at Mile Marker 1, State Highway 150, (505) 776-8787; as the name indicates, chile is the star.

Santa Fe possesses a number of fine Mexican eateries. **Tomasita's,** 500 South Guadaloupe Street, (505) 983-5721, features roast burrito with green chile and sour cream, carne avovada (pork marinated in red chiles), and a regional specialty—blue corn tortilla chips. **La Casa Sena,** 125 East Palace Avenue, (505) 988-9232, has singing waiters and waitresses in its cantina, which serves stuffed trout baked in clay. At **The Shed,** 113½ East Taos, a sign at the door proclaims: "Not responsible for Hot Chile."

Some readings to enhance travels: Dozier, Edward A., *The Pueblo Indians of North America,* Waveland Press, 1983; Edelman, Saundra A., *Summer People, Winter People: A Guide to the Pueblos in the Santa Fe Area,* Sunstone Press, 1986; Guthe, Carl E., *Pueblo Pottery Making: A Study of the Village of San Ildefonso,* AMS Press, 1981 (reprint of 1925 ed.); White, Leslie A., *Pueblo of San Felipe,* Kraus, (reprint of 1932 ed.). See also the readings for "Bat Flight Breakfast," page 200.

Turn off here along the way: To the Pueblo Indians of northern New Mexico, Santa Fe is a meeting place between their culture and the tourist trade. Their home is in the Rio Grande Valley near Espanola, between Santa Fe and Taos.

The **San Ildefonso Pueblo,** (505) 455-2273, is famous for its crafts, such as the pottery made by the renowned potter Maria Martinez. The pueblo is open to the public, but please note that you must pay a fee in order to take a photograph or paint. Pottery and painting are also part of the culture and economy of the **Santa Clara Pueblo,** (505) 753-7326, and the **San Juan Pueblo,** (505) 852-4400, two other pueblos located in Espanola.

There are a total of eight pueblos in the area. All of them hold their own feast days throughout the year. Call them to get accurate information about their schedules.

Santa Fe is a town full of history and culture. It dates back to 1610, when it was a Spanish provincial capital. The original plaza still exists and is the focal point for a number of museums and historic structures in a uniquely quaint atmosphere.

Event: Gold Rush Days
When: Early February
Where: Wickenburg, Arizona

Contact: Chamber of Commerce
Drawer CC
Wickenburg, AZ 85358
(602) 684-5479

Something about the event: The Wickenburg fairgrounds are the location for a three-day old-timers' rodeo, a Wild West parade, arts and crafts, and panning for gold.

Accommodations with a personal touch:
   Kay El Bar Ranch (R), Box 2480, Wickenburg, AZ 85358, (602) 684-7593: 10 rms, pb, $165-185 per week; cc-MC, V; c-yes, s-ltd, p-no, d-ltd, Full Bkfst; h-Jan Martin. Ranch is a National Historic Site, with adobe buildings. Full breakfasts and outdoor activities for the whole family.
   Bed and Breakfast in Arizona, Inc. (S), 8433 North Black Canyon Highway, Suite 160, Phoenix, AZ 85021, (602) 995-2831.

Roadside food: Anita's Casinas, 57 North Valentine Street, Wickenburg, (602) 684-5777, is a Mexican restaurant of distinction owned and run by one of Wickenburg's oldest families. Barbecue is cooked slowly in Chinese ovens at the **Frontier Inn**, 466 East Center Street, Wickenburg, (602) 684-2183.

Some readings to enhance travels: Fisher, Vardis, and Holmes, Opal L., *Gold Rushes and Mining Camps of the Early American West*, Carter, 1968; Pallatz, Harold, *The Gold Towns*, Ideal World, 1977; Robertson, Walter J., *Gold Panning for Profits*, Outbooks, 1978; Ransom, Jay E., *The Gold Hunter's Field Book: How and Where To Find Gold in the United States and Canada*, Harper & Row, 1980. See also "Cinco de Mayo," page 183.

Turn off here along the way: Wickenburg was settled in the 1860s for two reasons: One was gold,. the other water. The gold rush made Wickenburg Arizona's third largest city in 1866. More than $20 million in gold is said to have been carried from the nearby Vulture Mine. Wickenburg's river, the Hussayumpa, was dubbed "The River Flowing Upside Down" because the flow is 20 feet below ground.

The history of Wickenburg is explored at the **Desert Caballeros Western Museum,** North Frontier Street, (602) 684-2272. Exhibits include a re-creation of a Wickenburg street from the gold-rush era.

Former mining country extends to the north through communities such as **Yarnell, Prescott** and **Jerome.** Today, all have become prime getaway vacation destinations.

Event: Chinese New Year
When: February (varies with lunar calendar)
Where: San Francisco, California

Contact: San Francisco Visitor Information Center
P.O. Box 6977
San Francisco, CA 94101
(415) 391-2000

Something about the event: North America's foremost Chinese community salutes the New Year with pageants, cultural programs, lion dances, and the Golden Dragon Parade.

Accommodations with a personal touch:
Albion House (B&B), 135 Gough Street, San Francisco, CA 94102, (415) 621-0896: 8 rms, pb, $63-105; cc-AE, DC, MC, V; c-yes, s-yes, d-no, p-no, Cont Bkfst; h-Richard Meyer and Jeff Farris. Historic hotel, built in 1906, just after the earthquake in a former brothel district. Wood floors, stuffed pillows, atrium, fireplaces, antiques, and parlor piano.

The **Archbishop Mansion** (I), 1000 Fulton Street, San Francisco, CA 94117, (415) 563-7872: 15 rms, pb, $100-250; cc-AE, MC, V; c-ltd, s-ltd, d-no, p-no, Cont Bkfst; h-Ralph Woellmer. French-chateau-style inn facing Alamo Square Park was built in 1904 and survived the quake. Hand-carved mahogany, carved beds, chandeliers, and a jacuzzi are just some of the highlights.

The **Inn San Francisco** (I), 945 South Van Ness, San Francisco, CA 94114, (415) 641-0188: 15 rms, 12 pb, $60-160; cc-AE, MC, V;

c-over 12, s-yes, d-no, p-no, Cont Bkfst; h-Joel Daily. Mansion in historic Victorian district. Antiques, original woodwork, high ceilings, jacuzzi, and views.

Stanyan Park Hotel (H), 750 Stanyan Street, San Francisco, CA 94115, (415) 751-1000: 36 rms, pb, $62-145; cc-AE, DISC, MC, V; c-yes, s-yes, d-yes, p-no, Cont Bkfst. Long abandoned, this turn-of-the-century hotel has been restored and now features old-fashioned wallpaper, a sitting room, and a location near Golden Gate Park.

Roadside food: Restaurants throughout Chinatown offer specials for the Chinese New Year. In many places, there is entertainment as well. One such restaurant is **Yet Woh,** Pier 39, (415) 434-4430. It features Mandarin poultry and beef dishes and specializes in crab and lobster.

Italian cuisine is popular in San Francisco. **Washington Square Bar and Grill,** 1707 Powell Street, (415) 982-8123, specializes in pasta, veal, chicken, and seafood. Speaking of seafood, Fisherman's Wharf is the site of many legendary San Francisco seafood restaurants. One is **Tarantino's,** 206 Jefferson, (415) 839-4472.

Some readings to enhance travels: Kung, Shien-Woo, *Chinese in American Life,* Greenwood, 1973 (reprint of 1962 ed.); Chen, Jack, *The Chinese of America,* Harper & Row, 1982; Dicker, Laverne, *The Chinese in San Francisco: A Pictorial History,* Dover, 1980; Salter, Christopher L., *San Francisco's Chinatown: How Chinese a Town?,* R&E Publications, 1978.

Turn off here along the way: One of the best ways to get the feel for the largest Chinese city outside Asia is by walking through the 16 square blocks called **Chinatown.**

The main thoroughfare is Grant Avenue. There you'll see shops, temples, tea rooms, and a variety of businesses. It is, in fact, a self-contained community, commercially and financially.

The **Chinese Historical Society of America,** 17 Adler Place, (414) 391-1188, chronicles the history and culture of the Chinese in San Francisco. Chinese art and artifacts can be seen at the **Chinese Culture Center,** 250 Kearny Street, (415) 986-1822. Tours of Chinatown are available through the center.

San Francisco is also a locus of Japanese culture. The impact of transpacific trade can be seen at the **Japan Center,** 1520 Fillmore Street, (415) 922-6776. It is a complex that includes a hotel, consulate headquarters, offices, merchants, and a peace pagoda.

There is a Japanese tea garden in **Golden Gate Park.** It is a re-creation of a garden in Kyoto, Japan, and is surrounded by walks, waterfalls, cherry trees, and pagodas. Afternoon tea with an Asian flavor is served daily; call (415) 221-1311.

Angel Island, (415) 556-0560, was the equivalent of Ellis Island for Asian immigrants. A former military post and quarantine station, it is now a state park.

Of course, when you say "San Francisco," you're talking about the Golden Gate Bridge, Fisherman's Wharf, and the cable cars. You can take an unusually close look at the cable cars at the **Cable Car Museum,** Washington and Mason, (415) 474-1887. It displays models, pictures, the first cable car, and memorabilia of the history of this unique mode of ground transportation and its special place in San Francisco (see "Turning Back the Clock on American Transportation," page 137).

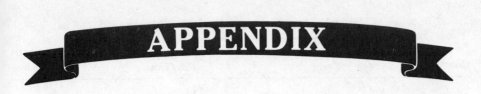

APPENDIX

Directory of Events by Month

Month	State	Event	City/Town	Page No.
January	AZ	Hopi Social Dances	Hopi Reservation	214
	CO	Western Stock Show	Denver	169
	ID	Basque Sheepherders' Ball and Lamb Auction	Boise	174
	MI	Polar Ice Cap Golf Tournament	Grand Haven	129
	NM	San Ildefonso Pueblo Feast Day	Pueblo Tribal Lands, Santa Fe	215
	NV	Cowboy Poetry Gathering	Elko	213
	PA	Mummers Parade	Philadelphia	47
	TX	Southwest Exposition Fat Stock Show and Rodeo	Fort Worth	172
	VA	Confederate Patriots' Birthdays	Lexington	91
	WI	Lakeside Winter Celebration	Fond du Lac	130
January–February	MN	St. Paul Winter Carnival	St. Paul	175
February	AZ	Gold Rush Days	Wickenburg	217
	CA	Chinese New Year	San Francisco	219
	PA	Groundhog Day	Punxsutawney	43
	PA	The Great American Chocolate Festival	Hershey	48
February–March	KS	International Pancake Race	Liberal	133
March	CA	Mendocino Coast Whale Festival	Mendocino–Fort Bragg	184
	MT	Western Art Auction	Great Falls	171
	OH	Buzzard Sunday	Hinckley	99
	VT	Town Meeting	Waitsfield	13
April	GA	Confederate Memorial Day	Atlanta	55

Directory of Events by Month

Month	State	Event	City/Town	Page No.
April	KY	Kentucky Derby Festival	Louisville	60
	MA	Patriots Day	Lexington	15
	MN	Festival of Nations	St. Paul	143
	MS	Catfish Capital of the World Festival	Belzoni	59
	NC	National Whistlers' Convention	Louisburg	57
	OK	89er Days	Guthrie	145
	UT	Anniversary of Golden Spike Ceremony	Promontory	140
	UT	Horseback Endurance Ride	Hurricane	141
	VT	Maple Sugar Festival	St. Albans	17
May	AZ	Cinco de Mayo	Nogales	183
	CA	Jumpin' Frog Jubilee	Angels Camp	188
	DC	Memorial Day	Washington, D.C.	11
	IN	500 Festival	Indianapolis	102
	MD	U.S. Naval Academy Commissioning Week	Annapolis	18
	MI	Tulip Time	Holland	100
	MO	Lewis and Clark Rendezvous	St. Charles	103
	MS	Jimmie Rodgers Memorial Festival	Meridian	62
	OR	Fleet of Flowers	Depoe Bay	190
	WA	Cherry Blossom and Japanese Culture Festival	Seattle	186
June	PA	Civil War Memorial	Gettysburg	26
June–July	MN	Sinclair Lewis Days	Sauk Centre	149
July	CA	Gilroy Garlic Festival	Gilroy	197
	CA	U.S. Open Sandcastle Competition	Imperial Beach	195
	DC	Independence Day in the Nation's Capital	Washington	27
	FL	Hemingway Days	Key West	73
	FL	Old-Fashioned Fourth of July	White Springs	71
	IL	Lincolnfest	Springfield	109
	IN	Oldest Consecutive Fourth of July Homecoming Celebration	Pekin	107
	ME	Maine Lobster Festival	Rockland	29
	MO	Tom Sawyer Days	Hannibal	110
	SC	Hillbilly Day	Mountain Rest	70
	UT	Days of '47 Pioneer Celebration	Salt Lake City	150

Directory of Events by Month

Month	State	Event	City/Town	Page No.
July	WI	The Great Circus Parade	Milwaukee	112
	WY	Frontier Days	Cheyenne	153
August	CO	State Fair (Colorado)	Pueblo	155
	IA	National Hobo Convention	Britt	114
	NC	Mountain Dance and Folk Festival	Asheville	68
	NM	Bat Flight Breakfast	Carlsbad	200
	NY	Baseball Hall of Fame Induction Ceremonies	Cooperstown	24
	TX	Texas Folklife Festival	San Antonio	152
	WA	Loggers' Jubilee	Morton	199
September	CA	Delicato Grape Stomp	Manteca	205
	ID	Idaho Spud Day	Shelley	159
	MI	Old Car Festival	Dearborn	120
	MS	Delta Blues Festival	Greenville	78
	TX	Republic of Texas Chilympiad	San Marcos	167
	WI	Wine and Harvest Festival	Cedarburg	122
September–October	VT	Vermont Fall Foliage Festival	Walden, Cabot, Plainfield, Peacham, Barnet, and Groton	35
October	IA	National Cornhusking Championship	Des Moines	119
	MA	Haunted Happenings	Salem	33
	MN	Norsfest and Lutefisk Day	Madison	162
	MT	Bison Roundup	Moiese	161
	NJ	Victorian Week	Cape May	37
	NM	Albuquerque International Balloon Fiesta	Albuquerque	207
	NY	World Pumpkin Federation Weigh-in	Collins	36
	OH	Circleville Pumpkin Show	Circleville	123
	TN	National Storytelling Festival	Jonesborough	77
	WA	Fall Foliage Festival	Leavenworth	209
	WA	Salmon Days	Issaquah	208
November	AR	World's Championship Duck-Calling Contest	Stuttgart	79
	IA	National Farm Toy Show	Dyersville	125
	MA	Plymouth Thanksgiving	Plymouth	39
	OK	Will Rogers Day	Claremore	164
	SC	Plantation Days	Charleston	81

Directory of Events by Month

Month	State	Event	City/Town	Page No.
December	AR	Ozark Christmas	Mountain View	90
	IN	Christmas Bird Count	Indiana Dunes	131
	LA	A Cajun Christmas	Lafayette	87
	MA	First Night	Boston	45
	NC	First Flight Commemoration	Kill Devil Hills	89

Directory of Events by State

State	Month	Event	City/Town	Page No.
AR	November	World's Championship Duck-Calling Contest	Stuttgart	79
	December	Ozark Christmas	Mountain View	90
AZ	January	Hopi Social Dances	Hopi Reservation	214
	February	Gold Rush Days	Wickenburg	217
	May	Cinco de Mayo	Nogales	183
CA	February	Chinese New Year	San Francisco	219
	March	Mendocino Coast Whale Festival	Mendocino–Fort Bragg	184
	May	Jumpin' Frog Jubilee	Angels Camp	188
	July	Gilroy Garlic Festival	Gilroy	197
	July	U.S. Open Sandcastle Competition	Imperial Beach	195
	September	Delicato Grape Stomp	Manteca	205
CO	January	Western Stock Show	Denver	169
	August	State Fair (Colorado)	Pueblo	155
DC	May	Memorial Day	Washington	11
	July	Independence Day in the Nation's Capital	Washington	27
FL	July	Hemingway Days	Key West	73
	July	Old-Fashioned Fourth of July	White Springs	71
GA	April	Confederate Memorial Day	Atlanta	55
IA	August	National Hobo Convention	Britt	114
	October	National Cornhusking Championship	Des Moines	119
	November	National Farm Toy Show	Dyersville	125
ID	January	Basque Sheepherders' Ball and Lamb Auction	Boise	174

Directory of Events by State

State	Month	Event	City/Town	Page No.
ID	September	Idaho Spud Day	Shelley	159
IL	July	Lincolnfest	Springfield	109
IN	May	500 Festival	Indianapolis	102
	July	Oldest Consecutive Fourth of July Homecoming Celebration	Pekin	107
	December	Christmas Bird Count	Indiana Dunes	131
KS	February–March	International Pancake Race	Liberal	133
KY	April	Kentucky Derby Festival	Louisville	60
LA	December	A Cajun Christmas	Lafayette	87
MA	April	Patriots Day	Lexington	15
	October	Haunted Happenings	Salem	33
	November	Plymouth Thanksgiving	Plymouth	39
	December	First Night	Boston	45
MD	May	U.S. Naval Academy Commissioning Week	Annapolis	18
ME	July	Maine Lobster Festival	Rockland	29
MI	January	Polar Ice Cap Golf Tournament	Grand Haven	129
	May	Tulip Time	Holland	100
	September	Old Car Festival	Dearborn	120
MN	January–February	St. Paul Winter Carnival	St. Paul	175
	April	Festival of Nations	St. Paul	143
	June–July	Sinclair Lewis Days	Sauk Centre	149
	October	Norsfest and Lutefisk Day	Madison	162
MO	May	Lewis and Clark Rendezvous	St. Charles	103
	July	Tom Sawyer Days	Hannibal	110
MS	April	Catfish Capital of the World Festival	Belzoni	59
	May	Jimmie Rodgers Memorial Festival	Meridian	62
	September	Delta Blues Festival	Greenville	78
MT	March	Western Art Auction	Great Falls	171
	October	Bison Roundup	Moiese	161
NC	April	National Whistlers' Convention	Louisburg	57
	August	Mountain Dance and Folk Festival	Asheville	68
	December	First Flight Commemoration	Kill Devil Hills	89
NJ	October	Victorian Week	Cape May	37

Directory of Events by State

State	Month	Event	City/Town	Page No.
NM	January	San Ildefonso Pueblo Feast Day	Pueblo Tribal Lands, Santa Fe	215
	August	Bat Flight Breakfast	Carlsbad	200
	October	Albuquerque International Balloon Fiesta	Albuquerque	207
NV	January	Cowboy Poetry Gathering	Elko	213
NY	August	Baseball Hall of Fame Induction Ceremonies	Cooperstown	24
	October	World Pumpkin Federation Weigh-in	Collins	36
OH	March	Buzzard Sunday	Hinckley	99
	October	Circleville Pumpkin Show	Circleville	123
OK	April	89er Days	Guthrie	145
	November	Will Rogers Day	Claremore	164
OR	May	Fleet of Flowers	Depoe Bay	190
PA	January	Mummers Parade	Philadelphia	47
	February	Groundhog Day	Punxsutawney	43
	February	The Great American Chocolate Festival	Hershey	48
	June	Civil War Memorial	Gettysburg	26
SC	July	Hillbilly Day	Mountain Rest	70
	November	Plantation Days	Charleston	81
TN	October	National Storytelling Festival	Jonesborough	77
TX	January	Southwest Exposition Fat Stock Show and Rodeo	Fort Worth	172
	August	Texas Folklife Festival	San Antonio	152
	September	Republic of Texas Chilympiad	San Marcos	167
UT	April	Anniversary of Golden Spike Ceremony	Promontory	140
	April	Horseback Endurance Ride	Hurricane	141
	July	Days of '47 Pioneer Celebration	Salt Lake City	150
VA	January	Confederate Patriots' Birthdays	Lexington	91
VT	March	Town Meeting	Waitsfield	99
	April	Maple Sugar Festival	St. Albans	17
	September–October	Vermont Fall Foliage Festival	Walden, Cabot, Plainfield, Peacham, Barnet, and Groton	35
WA	May	Cherry Blossom and	Seattle	

Directory of Events by State

State	Month	Event	City/Town	Page No.
WA		Japanese Culture Festival		186
	August	Loggers' Jubilee	Morton	199
	October	Fall Foliage Festival	Leavenworth	209
	October	Salmon Days	Issaquah	208
WI	January	Lakeside Winter Carnival	Fond du Lac	130
	July	The Great Circus Parade	Milwaukee	112
	September	Wine and Harvest Festival	Cedarburg	122
WY	July	Frontier Days	Cheyenne	153

Directory of Events by Type of Event

Description	Month	State	Event	City/Town	Page No.
Cultural/ Literary/ Music	March	MT	Western Art Auction	Great Falls	171
	May	MS	Jimmie Rodgers Memorial Festival	Meridian	62
	June–July	MN	Sinclair Lewis Days	Sauk Centre	149
	July	FL	Hemingway Days	Key West	73
	July	MO	Tom Sawyer Days	Hannibal	110
	September	MS	Delta Blues Festival	Greenville	78
	October	TN	National Storytelling Festival	Jonesborough	77
	November	OK	Will Rogers Day	Claremore	164
	December	MA	First Night	Boston	45
Ethnic	January	AZ	Hopi Social Dances	Hopi Reservation	214
	January	ID	Basque Sheepherders' Ball and Lamb Auction	Boise	174
	January	NM	San Ildefonso Pueblo Feast Day	Pueblo Tribal Lands, Santa Fe	215

Directory of Events by Type of Event

Description	Month	State	Event	City/Town	Page No.
Ethnic	February	CA	Chinese New Year	San Francisco	217
	April	MN	Festival of Nations	St. Paul	143
	May	AZ	Cinco de Mayo	Nogales	183
	May	WA	Cherry Blossom and Japanese Culture Festival	Seattle	186
	October	MN	Norsfest and Lutefisk Day	Madison	162
Folk	January	NV	Cowboy Poetry Gathering	Elko	213
	January	TX	Southwest Exposition Fat Stock Show and Rodeo	Fort Worth	172
	July	WY	Frontier Days	Cheyenne	153
	August	NC	Mountain Dance and Folk Festival	Asheville	68
	August	TX	Texas Folklife Festival	San Antonio	152
	August	WA	Loggers' Jubilee	Morton	199
	December	AR	Ozark Christmas	Mountain View	90
Food	February	PA	The Great American Chocolate Festival	Hershey	48
	April	MS	Catfish Capital of the World Festival	Belzoni	59
	July	CA	Gilroy Garlic Festival	Gilroy	197
	July	ME	Maine Lobster Festival	Rockland	29
	September	ID	Idaho Spud Day	Shelley	159
	September	TX	Republic of Texas Chilympiad	San Marcos	167
Historic	January	VA	Confederate Patriots' Birthdays	Lexington	91
	February	AZ	Gold Rush Days	Wickenburg	217
	March	VT	Town Meeting	Waitsfield	13
	April	GA	Confederate	Atlanta	

Directory of Events by Type of Event

Description	Month	State	Event	City/Town	Page No.
Historic			Memorial Day		55
	April	MA	Patriots Day	Lexington	15
	April	OK	89er Days	Guthrie	145
	April	UT	Anniversary of Golden Spike Ceremony	Promontory	140
	April	UT	Horseback Endurance Ride	Hurricane	141
	May	DC	Memorial Day	Washington	11
	May	MD	U.S. Naval Academy Commission-ing Week	Annapolis	18
	May	MO	Lewis and Clark Rendezvous	St. Charles	103
	May	OR	Fleet of Flowers	Depoe Bay	190
	June	PA	Civil War Memorial	Gettysburg	26
	July	DC	Independence Day in the Nation's Capital	Washington	27
	July	FL	Old-Fashioned Fourth of July	White Springs	71
	July	IL	Lincolnfest	Springfield	109
	July	IN	Oldest Consecutive Fourth of July Homecoming Celebration	Pekin	107
	July	SC	Hillbilly Day	Mountain Rest	70
	July	UT	Days of '47 Pioneer Celebration	Salt Lake City	150
	November	MA	Plymouth Thanksgiving	Plymouth	39
	December	NC	First Flight Commemora-tion	Kill Devil Hills	89
Rural/ Farm/ Nature	March	CA	Mendocino Coast Whale Festival	Mendocino– Fort Bragg	184
	March	OH	Buzzard Sunday	Hinckley	99
	April	VT	Maple Sugar Festival	St. Albans	17
	May	MI	Tulip Time	Holland	100

Directory of Events by Type of Event

Description	Month	State	Event	City/Town	Page No.
Rural/ Farm/ Nature	August	CO	State Fair (Colorado)	Pueblo	155
	August	NM	Bat Flight Breakfast	Carlsbad	200
	September–October	VT	Vermont Fall Foliage Festival	Walden, Cabot, Plainfield, Peacham, Barnet, and Groton	35
	October	IA	National Cornhusking Championship	Des Moines	119
	October	MT	Bison Roundup	Moiese	161
	October	NY	World Pumpkin Federation Weigh-in	Collins	36
	October	OH	Circleville Pumpkin Show	Circleville	123
	October	WA	Fall Foliage Festival	Leavenworth	209
	October	WA	Salmon Days	Issaquah	208
	November	SC	Plantation Days	Charleston	81
	December	IN	Christmas Bird Count	Indiana Dunes	131
Seasonal	January	WI	Lakeside Winter Carnival	Fond du Lac	130
	January–February	MN	St. Paul Winter Carnival	St. Paul	175
	September	CA	Delicato Grape Stomp	Manteca	205
	September	WI	Wine and Harvest Festival	Cedarburg	122
	December	LA	A Cajun Christmas	Lafayette	87
Miscellaneous	January	CO	Western Stock Show	Denver	169
	January	MI	Polar Ice Cap Golf Tournament	Grand Haven	129
	January	PA	Mummers Parade	Philadelphia	47
	February	PA	Groundhog Day	Punxsutawney	43
	February–March	KS	International Pancake Race	Liberal	133

Directory of Events by Type of Event

Description	Month	State	Event	City/Town	Page No.
Miscellaneous	April	KY	Kentucky Derby and Festival	Louisville	60
	April	NC	National Whistlers' Convention	Louisburg	57
	May	CA	Jumpin' Frog Jubilee	Angels Camp	188
	May	IN	500 Festival	Indianapolis	102
	July	CA	U.S. Open Sandcastle Competition	Imperial Beach	195
	July	WI	The Great Circus Parade	Milwaukee	112
	August	IA	National Hobo Convention	Britt	114
	August	NY	Baseball Hall of Fame Induction Ceremonies	Cooperstown	24
	September	MI	Old Car Festival	Dearborn	120
	October	MA	Haunted Happenings	Salem	33
	October	NJ	Victorian Week	Cape May	37
	October	NM	Albuquerque International Balloon Fiesta	Albuquerque	207
	November	AR	World's Championship Duck-Calling Contest	Stuttgart	79
	November	IA	National Farm Toy Show	Dyersville	125

Directory of Accommodations by State

State	Inn	City/Town	Type	Budget*	Page No.
AR	Commercial Hotel on the Square	Mountain View	Hotel	m	90
	Edwardian Inn	Helena	Inn	m	80
	Inn of Mountain View B&B	Mountain View	Inn	m	90
	Margland II	Pine Bluff	Inn	m	80
	The Great Southern Hotel	Brinkley	Hotel	m	80
AZ	Arizona Inn	Tucson	Hotel	m,d	183
	Bed & Breakfast in Arizona	Phoenix	Service	b,m,d	183, 217
	Dierker House	Flagstaff	B&B	b,m	214
	Hacienda del Sol	Tucson	Hotel	b,m,d	183
	Kay El Bar Ranch	Wickenburg	Ranch	m	217
	Mi Casa Su Casa Bed & Breakfast	Tempe	Service	b,m,d	183
	Walking L Ranch	Flagstaff	Ranch	b,m	214
CA	Albion House	San Francisco	Hotel	m,d	218
	Ambert House	Sacramento	Inn	m,d	205
	Aunt Abigail's B&B	Sacramento	Inn	m	205
	Babbling Brook Inn	Santa Cruz	Inn	d	197
	Bayview Hotel	Aptos	Hotel	m	197
	Bear Flag Inn	Sacramento	Inn	m	205
	Briggs House	Sacramento	Inn	m,d	205
	Britt House	San Diego	Inn	d	195
	Carolyn's Bed & Breakfast Homes in San Diego	San Diego	Service	b,m,d	196
	Country Inn	Fort Bragg	Inn	m,d	185
	Darling House	Santa Cruz	Inn	m,d	198
	Dunbar House	Murphys	Inn	m	188
	Harbor Hill Guest House	San Diego	B&B	m	195
	Heritage Park Bed & Breakfast	San Diego	Inn	d	195
	Joshua Grindle Inn	Mendocino	Inn	m,d	185
	Mangels House	Aptos	Inn	d	197
	Mendocino Village Bed & Breakfast	Mendocino	Inn	m,d	185
	Murphys Hotel	Murphys	Hotel	m	188
	Stanyan Park Hotel	San Francisco	Inn	m,d	219
	Sutter Creek Inn	Sutter Creek	Hotel	m	188
	The Archbishop Mansion	San Francisco	Inn	d	218

*b–budget, m–moderate, d–deluxe

Directory of Accommodations by State

State	Inn	City/Town	Type	Budget*	Page No.
CA	The Grey Whale Inn	Fort Bragg	Inn	m,d	185
	The Inn San Francisco	San Francisco	Inn	m,d	218
CO	Bed & Breakfast Colorado	Denver	Service	b,m,d	170
	Bed & Breakfast Rocky Mountains	Colorado Springs	Service	b,m,d	155, 171
	Oxford Hotel	Denver	Hotel	m	169
	The Brown Palace	Denver	Hotel	d	169
	The Dove Inn	Golden	Inn	m	169
	The Heatherstone Inn	Colorado Springs	Inn	m,d	155
DC	Adams Inn	Washington	Inn	m	11
	Kalorama Guest House–Woodley	Washington	Inn	m	11
	Kalorama Guest House–Kalorama	Washington	Inn	m	11
	Swiss Inn	Washington	Hotel	m	11
	The Jefferson Hotel	Washington	Hotel	m,d	11
	Willard Hotel	Washington	Hotel	d	11
FL	B&B on the Ocean	Big Pine Key	Inn	m	73
	Bed & Breakfast of the Florida Keys	Winter Park	Service	b,m,d	73
	Casa De Solana	St. Augustine	B&B	d	71
	Hopp Inn Guest House	Marathon	B&B	m	73
	Suncoast Accommodations	St. Petersburg	Service	b,m,d	71
	Susina Plantation Inn	Thomasville	Inn	d	71
	The Kenwood	St Augustine	Inn	m	71
	The Wicker Guest House	Key West	B&B	m,d	73
GA	Arden Hall	Marietta	Inn	m	56
	Bed & Breakfast– Atlanta	Atlanta	Service	b,m,d	56
	Beverly Hills Inn	Atlanta	Inn	m,d	56
	The Culpepper House	Senoia	Inn	b,m	55
IA	Bed & Breakfast in Iowa	Des Moines	Service	b,m,d	114, 125
	Heritage House	Leighton	B&B	m	119
	Hotel Brooklyn	Brooklyn	Inn	b	119
	Redstone Inn	Dubuque	Inn	d	125
	Stout House	Dubuque	B&B	m	125

Directory of Accommodations by State

State	Inn	City/Town	Type	Budget*	Page No.
IA	Walden Acres	Adel	B&B	m	119
ID	Idaho City Hotel	Idaho City	Hotel	b,m	174
	Pensione Hermaine	Blackfoot	Inn	b,m	159
IL	Hamilton House	Springfield	B&B	m	109
	Mischler House	Springfield	B&B	m	109
IN	Creekwood Inn	Michigan City	Inn	d	132
	Duneland Inn	Michigan City	Inn	m,d	132
	Hollingsworth House Inn	Indianapolis	Inn	m,d	102
	Plantation Inn	Michigan City	Inn	m,d	132
	The Cliff House	Madison	B&B	m	108
	The Pairadux Inn	Indianapolis	Inn	m	102
	Ye Old Scotts Inn	Leavenworth	Inn	b	108
KS	Cimarron Hotel & Restaurant	Cimarron	Hotel	b,m	133
	Hardesty House	Ashland	Inn	b	133
KY	Kentucky Homes Bed & Breakfast	Louisville	Service	b,m,d	60
KY	Log Cabin Bed & Breakfast	Georgetown	B&B	m	60
	Seebach Hotel	Louisville	Hotel	d	60
LA	Bois des Chenes Plantation	Lafayette	Inn	m,d	87
	Ti Frere's House	Lafayette	B&B	m	87
MA	Amelia Payson Guest House	Salem	Inn	m	33
	Be Our Guest Bed & Breakfast	Plymouth	Service	b,m,d	39
	Chandler Inn	Boston	Inn	m	45
	Colonial House Inn	Plymouth	Inn	m	39
	Copley Plaza Hotel	Boston	Hotel	d	45
	Greater Boston Hospitality	Brookline	Service	b,m,d	46
	John Ashley Bed & Breakfast	Lexington	B&B	m	15
	Morton Park Place	Plymouth	B&B	m	39
	Ritz Carlton Hotel	Boston	Hotel	d	45
	Salem Inn	Salem	Inn	m,d	33
	Stephen Daniels House	Salem	Inn	m	33
	Sterling Inn	Sterling	Inn	m,d	15
	The Coach House Inn	Salem	Inn	m	33
	The Hawthorne Inn	Concord	Inn	d	15
MD	Gibson's Lodgings	Annapolis	Inn	m,d	18

*b–budget, m–moderate, d–deluxe

Directory of Accommodations by State

State	Inn	City/Town	Type	Budget*	Page No.
MD	Governor Calvert House	Annapolis	Inn	d	18
	Maryland Inn	Annapolis	Inn	m,d	19
	Naomi Reed Inn	Annapolis	B&B	b	19
	Prince Johnson House	Annapolis	Inn	m	19
	Robert Johnson House	Annapolis	Inn	d	18
ME	Godspeed's Guest House	Camden	Inn	m	29
	The Belmont	Camden	Inn	m,d	29
	The Swan House	Camden	Inn	m,d	29
	Whitehall Inn	Camden	Inn	m,d	29
MI	Barclay Inn	Birmingham	Hotel	m,d	121
	Bed & Breakfast of Grand Rapids	Grand Rapids	Service	b,m,d	101
	Betsy Ross Bed & Breakfast	Bloomfield Hills	Service	b,m,d	121
	Blanche House Inn	Detroit	Inn	m	120
	Dearborn Inn	Dearborn	Hotel	m,d	120
	Old Wing Inn	Holland	Inn	m	101
	Twin Gables	Saugatuck	Inn	m	101
	Wickwood Inn	Saugatuck	Inn	d	101
MN	Bed & Breakfast Registry	St. Paul	Service	b,m,d	163
	Bed & Breakfast Upper Midwest	Crystal Lake	Service	b,m,d	163
	Chatsworth B&B	St Paul	B&B	m	143
	Nicolett Island Inn	Nicolett Island	Inn	m	143
	Palmer House Hotel	Sauk Centre	Hotel	b,m	149
	River Town Inn	Stillwater	Inn	m	143
	St. Paul Hotel	St. Paul	Hotel	d	143
	Thorwood	Hastings	Inn	m,d	143
MO	Bed & Breakfast of St. Louis, River Country of Missouri & Illinois	St. Louis	Service	b,m,d	103,110
	Fifth Street Mansion	Hannibal	Inn	m	110
	Schewegmann House	Washington	Inn	m	103
	The Victorian Guest House	Hannibal	B&B	b	110
MS	Anchua	Vicksburg	Inn	m,d	59
	Cedar Grove Inn	Vicksburg	Inn	m,d	59

Directory of Accommodations by State

State	Inn	City/Town	Type	Budget*	Page No.
MS	Grey Oaks	Vicksburg	Inn	m	59
	Lincoln Ltd. B&B	Meridian	Service	b,m,d	59, 62
MT	Murphy's House B&B	Great Falls	B&B	m	171
	Three Pheasant Inn	Great Falls	B&B	m	171
	Western Bed & Breakfast Hosts	Kalispell	Service	b,m	161, 171
NC	Albemarle Inn	Asheville	Inn	m	68
	Baird House Country Inn	Asheville	Inn	m	68
	Cedar Crest Victorian Inn	Asheville	Inn	m,d	68
	Crotan Inn/ Papagayo	Kill Devil Hills	Inn	b,m	89
	Duttonwood Inn	Franklin	Inn	m	70
	Flint Street Inn	Asheville	Inn	m	68
	Kings Arm Inn	New Bern	Inn	m	57
	Oakwood Inn	Raleigh	Inn	m	57
	Old Reynolds Mansion	Asheville	Inn	m	68
	Scarborough Inn	Manteo	Inn	b,m	89
	Summit Inn	Franklin	Inn	m	70
	The Old Edwards Inn	Highlands	Inn	m	70
	Ye Old Cherokee Inn	Kill Devil Hills	Inn	m	89
NJ	The Abbey	Cape May	Inn	m,d	37
	The Chalfonte Hotel	Cape May	Hotel	m,d	37
	The Mainstay	Cape May	Inn	m,d	37
	The Queen Victoria	Cape May	Inn	m,d	38
NM	Apple Tree Inn	Albuquerque	Inn	m,d	207
	Casita Chamisa	Albuquerque	B&B	m,d	207
	La Posada de Chimago	Chimago	Inn	m	215
	Orange Street Bed & Breakfast	Los Alamos	Inn	b	216
	The Lodge	Cloudcroft	Inn	m,d	200
NV	Breitenstein House	Lamoille	B&B	m	213
	Old Pioneer Garden	Unionville	Inn	m	213
NY	Cooper Inn	Cooperstown	Inn	m,d	24
	Grape Country Manor	Silver Creek	B&B	b,m	36
	Hickory Grove Inn	Cooperstown	Inn	m	24
	The Teepee	Gowanda	B&B	b	36
	Tunnicliff Inn	Cooperstown	Inn	m	24

*b–budget, m–moderate, d–deluxe

Directory of Accommodations by State

State	Inn	City/Town	Type	Budget*	Page No.
OH	B&B of Hocking County	Logan	Service	b,m,d	123
	Brandywine Inn	Sagamore	Inn	m,d	99
	Buckeye Bed & Breakfast	Powell	Service	b,m,d	99
	Colonial Manor Bed & Breakfast	Seville	B&B	b	99
	Waynesville Guest Haus	Waynesville	B&B	m	123
OK	Country Inn Bed & Breakfast	Claremore	B&B	m	164
	Flora's B&B	Oklahoma City	B&B	b	145
	The Grandison	Oklahoma City	Inn	b,m	145
	Will Rogers Hotel	Claremore	Hotel	m,d	164
OR	Channel House	Depoe Bay	Inn	m,d	190
	Northwest Bed & Breakfast	Portland	Service	b,m,d	174, 190
	Ocean House	Newport	B&B	m	190
PA	Appleford Inn	Gettysburg	Inn	m,d	26
	Bed & Breakfast in the Lancaster, Harrisburg & Hershey Areas	Elizabethtown	Service	b,m,d	48
	Bed & Breakfast of Philadelphia	Philadelphia	Service	b,m,d	47
	Bishop's Rocking Horse Inn	Gettysburg	Inn	d	26
	Gateway Lodge	Cooksburg	Inn	b	44
	Hotel Hershey	Hershey	Hotel	D	48
	Latham Hotel	Philadelphia	Hotel	D	47
	Rest & Repast B&B Service	Pine Grove	Service	b,m	44
	Society Hill Hotel	Philadelphia	Inn	D	47
	The Brafferton	Gettysburg	Inn	m	26
	The House of Serian	Punxsutawney	Inn	m	44
	Watsamatter Farm	Halifax	Farm	b	48
SC	Battery Carriage House	Charleston	Inn	d	81
	Elliot House Inn	Charleston	Inn	d	81
	Planters Inn	Charleston	Inn	d	81
	Two Meeting Place	Charleston	Inn	m,d	81
	Vendue Inn	Charleston	Inn	m,d	81
TN	Big Springs Inn	Greenville	Inn	m	77
	Hale Springs Inn	Rogersville	Inn	m	77
	Jonesborough Bed & Breakfast	Jonesborough	Service	b,m,d	77

Directory of Accommodations by State

State	Inn	City/Town	Type	Budget*	Page No.
TX	Aquarena Springs Inn	San Marcos	Inn	m	160
	Bed & Breakfast of San Antonio Home Lodging Service	San Antonio	Service	b,m,d	152
	Bed & Breakfast of Wimberly	Wimberly	Service	b,m,d	160
	Bed & Breakfast Texas Style	Dallas	Service	b,m,d	173
	Crystal River Inn	San Marcos	Inn	m	160
	Hotel Crescent Court	Dallas	Hotel	d	173
	Melrose Hotel	Dallas	Hotel	m,d	173
	Menger Hotel	San Antonio	Hotel	m,d	152
	Stockyards Hotel	Fort Worth	Hotel	d	173
	The Bullis	San Antonio	Hotel	b,m	152
UT	Center Street Bed & Breakfast	Logan	Inn	b,m	140
	Green Gate Village Bed & Breakfast	St. George	Inn	m,d	141
	National Historic Bed & Breakfast	Salt Lake City	Inn	m	150
	Pinecrest B&B Inn	Salt Lake City	Inn	m,d	150
	Saltair Bed & Breakfast	Salt Lake City	Inn	b,m	150
	Seven Wives Inn	St. George	Inn	b,m	141
	The Bed & Breakfast Association of Utah	Salt Lake City	Service	b,m,d	140
	The Bed & Breakfast Homestay of Utah	Salt Lake City	Service	b,m,d	150
	The Spruces B&B	Salt Lake City	B&B	m	150
	Under the Eaves Guest House	Springdale	B&B	b,m	141
	Zion House Bed & Breakfast	Springdale	B&B	b,m	141
VA	Alexander-Withe	Lexington	Inn	m	92
	Maple Hall	Lexington	Inn	m	92
	McCampbell House	Lexington	Inn	m,d	92
VT	Berkson Farms	Enosburg Falls	Farm	b,m	17

*b–budget, m–moderate, d–deluxe

Directory of Accommodations by State

State	Inn	City/Town	Type	Budget*	Page No.
VT	Highland Lodge	Greensboro	Inn	m,d	35
	Johnson House	Essex Junction	B&B	m	
	Knoll Country Inn	Waitsfield	Inn	b,m	17
	Lareau Farm				13
	Country Inn	Waitsfield	Inn	b,m	
	Mountain View Inn	Waitsfield	Inn	m	13
	Nutmaker Inn	East Burke	B&B	b	13
	Rabbit Hill Inn	Lower	Inn	b,m	35
		Wareford			35
	Tucker Hill Lodge	Waitsfield	Inn	m	
	Waitsfield Inn	Waitsfield	Inn	m,d	13
WA	Brown's Farm	Leavenworth	Farm	m	13
	Colonial Inn	Fall City	Inn	b,m	210
	Galer Place	Seattle	B&B	m	208
	Haus Rohrbach				186
	Pension	Leavenworth	Inn	m	210
	MV Challenger	Seattle	B&B	m	188
	National Park Inn	Longmire	Inn	m	199
	Pacific Bed &	Seattle	Service	b,m,d	187
	Sorrento Hotel	Seattle	Hotel	d	187
	The Wildflower	Issaquah	B&B	m	209
	Travelers Bed &				
	Breakfast	Mercer Island	Service	b,m,d	210
	Williams House	Seattle	Inn	m	186
WI	Bed & Breakfast of				
	Milwaukee	Milwaukee	Service	b,m,d	112
	Clarion Hotel	Fond du Lac	Hotel	m	130
	Deorshel's Bed &	Menomonee			
	Breakfast	Falls	B&B	m	112
	Hebbring Falls	Menomonee	Hotel	b,m	112
		Falls			
	Phister Inn	Milwaukee	Hotel	d	112
	Stage Coach Inn	Cedarburg	Inn	m	112
	The Farmer's				
	Daughter	Ripon	Inn	m	130
	Washington House				
	Inn	Cedarburg	Inn	m,d	112
WY	Two Bars Seven				
	Ranch	Tie Siding	Ranch	m	154
	Bed & Breakfast				
	Rocky Mountain	Cheyenne	Service	b,m,d	154

Bed and Breakfast Resources

National Services

American Bed and Breakfast Association
P.O. Box 23294
Washington, D.C. 20026
(202) 237-9777

Bed and Breakfast Reservation Services
125 Newton Road
Springfield, MA 01118
(413) 783-5111

The Bed and Breakfast League, Ltd.
2855 29th Street, N.W.
Washington, DC 20008
(202) 232-8718

Bed and Breakfast Hospitality
823 La Mirada Avenue
Leucadia, CA 92024

Home Suite Homes
1470 Firebird Way
Sunnyvale, CA 94087
(408) 733-7215

New Age Travel
P.O. Box 378
Encinitas, CA 92024
(619) 436-9977

Northwest Bed and Breakfast
7707 Southwest Locust Street
Portland, OR 97223
(503) 246-8366

O.T.R. Travel Information Servic[e]
P.O. Box 4262
River Edge, NJ 07661
(201) 487-1190

P.T. International
1318 Southwest Troy Street
Portland, OR 97219
(800) 547-1436, (503) 245-0440

Bed and Breakfast International
151 Ardmore Road
Kensington, CA 94707
(415) 525-45690

Bed and Breakfast Registry
P.O. Box 80174
St. Paul, MN 55108
(612) 646-4238

Bed and Breakfast Society
330 West Main Street
Fredericksburg, TX 78624
(512) 997-4712

Bed and Breakfast U.S.A., Ltd.
49 Van Wyck Street
New York, NY 10520
(914) 271-6228

Bed and Breakfast Books

Chesler, Bernice. *Bed and Breakfast Coast to Coast.* Lexington, MA: The Stephen Greene Press, 1986.

Christopher, Bob and Ellen. *Christopher's Bed and Breakfast Guide.* Millford, CT: Robert and Ellen Christopher, 1983.

Crosete, Barbara, and Wendy Lowe. *America's Wonderful Little Hotels and Inns.* New York: Congdon & Weed, Inc., 1986.

Dickerman, Pat. *Farm, Ranch and Country Vacations.* New York: Farm and Ranch Vacations, 1986.

Featherstone, Phyllis, and Barbara F. Ostler. *The Bed and Breakfast Guide.* Washington D.C.: National Bed and Breakfast Association, 1983.

Gieseling, Hal. *Frommer's Bed and Breakfast, North America.* New York: Simon & Schuster, Inc., 1986.

Hitchcock, Anthony, and Jean Lindgen. *Country Inns.* New York: Burt Franklin & Co, Inc., 1986. Series.

Lanier, Pamela. *The Complete Guide to Bed and Breakfasts, Inns and Guesthouses.* Santa Fe, NM: John Muir Press, 1986.

Notarius, Barbara. *The Bed & Breakfast Directory.* New York: John Wiley & Sons, Inc., 1988.

Ross, Corine Madden. *Bed and Breakfast.* Charlotte, NC: East Wood Press, 1986. Regional series.

Roundback, Betty Revits, and Nancy Kramer. *Bed and Breakfast, U.S.A.,* New York: EP Dutton, Inc., 1986.

Simpson, Norman T. *Bed and Breakfast American Style.* New York: Harper & Row, Publishers, Inc., 1987.

Thaxton, John. *Bed and Breakfast America.* New York: Burt Franklin & Co, Inc., 1985.

A Treasury of Bed and Breakfasts. Washington D.C.: American Bed and Breakfast Association, 1984.

Background Reading

American Association for State and Local History. *A Historical Guide to the United States.* New York: WW Norton & Co, Inc., 1986.

Brownstone, Douglass L. *A Field Guide to America's History.* New York: Facts on File Publications, 1984.

Chambers, S. Allen, ed. *Discovering Historic America.* New York: EP Dutton, Inc., 1982. Series.

Conrad, Peter. *Imagining America.* New York: Avon Books, 1980.

Cooke, Alistair. *The Americans.* New York: Alfred A. Knopf, Inc., 1979.

Cooke, Alistair. *Images of America.* New York: Alfred A. Knopf, Inc., 1977.

Fussell, Betty. *I Hear America Cooking.* New York: Viking Penguin, Inc., 1986.

Garreau, Joel. *The Nine Nations of North America.* Boston: Houghton Mifflin Co., 1981.

Geffen, Alica, and Carole Berglie. *Food Festival.* New York: Pantheon Books Inc., 1986.

Hendrickson, Robert. *America Talk, The Words and Ways of American Dialects.* New York: Viking Penguin, Inc., 1986.

Hogarth, Hugh. *The Golden Land.* New York: Pantheon Books, Inc., 1976.

Journonoy, Joyce, and David Jenness. *America on Display.* New York: Facts on File Publications, 1987.

Kuralt, Charles. *Dateline America.* New York: Harcourt Brace Jovanovich, Inc., 1979.

Kuralt, Charles. *On the Road with Charles Kuralt.* New York: The Putnam Publishing Group, Inc., 1984.

Malcom, Andrew H. *Unknown America.* New York: Times Books, 1975.

O'Neill, Thomas, and Ira Block. *Back Roads America.* Washington D.C.: National Geographic Society, 1980.

Patton, Phil. *Open Road: A Celebration of the American Highway.* New York: Simon & Schuster, Inc., 1986.

Pearce, Neil R., and Jerry Hagstrom. *The Book of America: Inside the 50 States Today.* New York: WW Norton & Co, Inc., 1983.

Simony, Maggy, ed. *The Traveler's Reading Guide.* New York: Facts on File Publications, 1987.

Stegner, Wallace and Page. *American Places.* New York: EP Dutton Inc., 1982.

Steinbeck, John. *Travels with Charley in Search of America.* New York: Bantam Books, Inc., 1977.

Stern, Jane and Michael. *Roadfood and Goodfood.* New York: Alfred A. Knopf, Inc., 1986.

Terkel, Studs. *American Dreams: Lost and Found.* New York: Pantheon Books, Inc., 1980.

Theroux, Paul. *The Old Patagonian Express: By Train through the Americas.* Boston: Houghton Mifflin Co., 1979.

USA Today Travel Tips. Kansas City and New York: Andrews, McMeel & Parker, 1987.

Weiner, Neal O., and David Schwartz. *The Interstate Gourmet.* New York: Summit Books, 1986.

Woodson, LeRoy, Jr. *Roadside Food: Good Home Style Cooking across America.* New York: Stewart, Tabori and Chang, 1986.

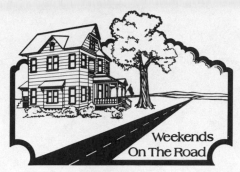

Weekends
On The Road

The Hidden America . . . . . continuing the journey

Friends:

Beyond the Interstate is but a starting point (and a small one) in unveiling the Hidden America.

Weekends on the Road offers a variety of subscriptions and memberships to help make this Hidden America accessible to travelers. They include events listings, publications, periodicals, and features on back-roads America.

We can help you discover where to find events such as the Republic of Texas Chilympiad, the Maine Lobster Festival, and the Jumpin' Frog Jubilee, and tell you what it's like there. In addition, our listings include cultural events in music, art, and theater. Events in Canada are covered too.

Our events and features can help you get out on the road, and they'll entertain you even if you can't get away from home.

We hope you decide to join with us as we continue our journey across America.

Your friends at
WEEKENDS ON THE ROAD

WEEKENDS ON THE ROAD is a one-stop source of information about hundreds of annual festivals and events, including lists of nearby accommodations with a personal touch and suggested readings. Membership includes newsletters and monthly events updates. Separate membership for *Weekends On The Road—Canada.* (SUBSCRIPTION PRICE—$25 U.S. for one year; $30 Canadian.)

For more information:
Write: P.O. Box 4262
River Edge, NJ 07661
Phone: (201) 487-1190 (New Jersey)

....

Name _____

Address _____

City _____

State _____ **Zip** _____

Phone _____

Subscription chosen

____ Weekends on the Road   ____ Weekends on the Road—Canada

Amount enclosed $_____
(Make checks payable to Weekends on the Road)